The Object Relations Lens

A Psychodynamic Framework
for the
Beginning Therapist

The Object Relations Lens

A Psychodynamic Framework
for the
Beginning Therapist

Christopher W. T. Miller, M.D.

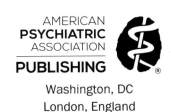

AMERICAN
PSYCHIATRIC
ASSOCIATION
PUBLISHING®

Washington, DC
London, England

If you wish to buy 50 or more copies of the same title, please go to www.appi.org/specialdiscounts for more information.

Copyright © 2023 American Psychiatric Association Publishing

ALL RIGHTS RESERVED

First Edition

Manufactured in the United States of America on acid-free paper
26   25   24   23   22   5   4   3   2   1

American Psychiatric Association Publishing
800 Maine Avenue SW, Suite 900
Washington, DC 20024-2812
www.appi.org

Library of Congress Cataloging-in-Publication Data
Names: Miller, Christopher W.T., author. | American Psychiatric Association, issuing body.
Title: The object relations lens : a psychodynamic framework for the beginning therapist / Christopher W.T. Miller.
Description: First edition. | Washington, DC : American Psychiatric Association Publishing, [2023] | Includes bibliographical references and index.
Identifiers: LCCN 2022019804 (print) | LCCN 2022019805 (ebook) | ISBN 9781615374281 (paperback) | ISBN 9781615374298 (ebook).
Subjects: MESH: Object Attachment | Psychotherapy, Psychodynamic | Professional-Patient Relations | Oedipus Complex.
Classification: LCC RC480.5 (print) | LCC RC480.5 (ebook) | NLM WM 460.5.O2 | DDC 616.89/14—dc23/eng/20220527.
LC record available at https://lccn.loc.gov/2022019804.
LC ebook record available at https://lccn.loc.gov/2022019805.

British Library Cataloguing in Publication Data
A CIP record is available from the British Library.

To my parents, with gratitude.

Contents

About the Author

Dr. Christopher W. T. Miller is an Associate Professor in the Department of Psychiatry at the University of Maryland School of Medicine. He obtained his medical degree from the Universidade Federal de Santa Catarina, in Florianópolis, Brazil. He trained in Adult Psychiatry at the University of Maryland/Sheppard Pratt Residency Program. He completed training in Adult Psychoanalysis at the Washington Baltimore Center for Psychoanalysis. He is the Director of Psychotherapy Education for the University of Maryland/Sheppard Pratt Psychiatry Residency Program. In addition to seeing patients for psychodynamic psychotherapy and psychoanalysis, he works in the Psychiatric Emergency Services. He has published and lectured on educational frameworks for teaching psychotherapy in residency programs, the intersection between the neurosciences and psychotherapy, and psychodynamic dimensions of film and literature. He lives in Baltimore, Maryland.

Foreword

FORTY YEARS AGO, I started seeing outpatients for psychotherapy. I was a third-year psychiatry resident, anxious and clueless. My only experience of psychotherapy was as a patient. It was then that I decided to add a psychotherapy book to my bedside table, alongside a novel and general nonfiction book. Every night, I read a chapter or two from one of them. Over time, I gained in experience as a therapist, and my anxiety subsided. I learned from my patients and supervisors. I kept reading. I undertook psychoanalytic training and kept reading. I became a psychotherapy supervisor, teacher, director of psychotherapy education, and director of residency training. As time rolled on, I taught several generations of psychiatry residents and psychoanalytic candidates. For 40 years, I kept reading novels, general nonfiction, and psychotherapy books with discipline and growing sophistication. I read more than 75 psychotherapy books in that time.

What is it about this book by Dr. Christopher Miller that sets it apart? Let me state three points.

First, it is an undeniable fact that this book is very well written. Dr. Miller is a gifted author and craftsman of the English language. He avoids unnecessary jargon and defines and elaborates difficult psychoanalytic concepts (such as projective identification) with admirable clarity. Theoretical points are carefully explained and then come to life with detailed clinical vignettes from his practice. This book is engaging, at times quite entertaining, and always relevant. Once you start it, you will finish it.

My second point is that this book is a rare combination of relevance, breadth, and depth. Although written for early career psychotherapists (and in particular psychiatric residents), it has much to offer a more seasoned reader. Dr. Miller speaks from the position of a clinician entering his prime, with real wisdom to share. He works in a variety of clinical settings, shoulder to shoulder with the young clinicians he trains. He has designed and refined a model curriculum on psychodynamic psychotherapy for third-year psychiatric residents that he uses to teach. This has helped him to be incisive in his thinking and writing. He supervises residents in their outpatient clinics and in the psychiatric emergency department. This has refined his mastery of the clinical material. He is up to date and expert in areas directly related to psychotherapy, such as neuroscience and sociocultural competencies. (If you question this, read Chapter 10 on the neuroscience of psychotherapy, which is a remarkable tour de force.) In addition to being contemporary, Dr. Miller is a true Renaissance man, which adds nuance and color to this book. For example, he is a self-educated Shakespeare scholar of some note. At key times, he brings in wisdom from literary sources to emphasize a clinical point. In sum, he knows his material, knows what trainees need to hear, and knows how to say it.

My third and final point involves the fundamental coherence of this psychotherapy text. It is a tremendous asset that this book has one author, presenting a single, consistent voice. Furthermore, it is grounded on one particular orientation of dynamic psychotherapy: object relations theory as developed by Melanie Klein and the modern Kleinian school. Theory, practical advice, and illustrative clinical material are integrated and reflected through the mind of one (very talented) clinician. They fit into a coherent whole. The student gets to sit on the shoulder of Dr. Miller and see how he thinks, what he feels, what he says, and how he acts with his patients in the office and in the emergency department.

In conclusion, Dr. Miller's book is an important addition to the literature on thinking from a psychodynamic perspective, practicing psychotherapy, and teaching this science and art to trainees. It is well worth reading, digesting, and incorporating into the psychotherapy practice of any clinician. It will prove especially useful to new therapists and supervisors alike.

Donald R. Ross, M.D.
Medical Director and Senior Psychiatrist (Emeritus),
The Retreat at Sheppard Pratt;
Training and Supervising Analyst,
The Washington-Baltimore Psychoanalytic Institute;
Clinical Associate Professor of Psychiatry (Emeritus),
University of Maryland School of Medicine

Introduction

The renowned monk Hakuin had a favorite expression that meditation in the midst of activity was far better than meditation in silence.

Andrew Juniper (2003, p. 26)

SOME YEARS AGO I was driving to Philadelphia to watch *The Turin Horse*, a film by Hungarian director Béla Tarr. One of the few twenty-first-century filmmakers to create long, black-and-white, meditative works, his films are unflinching portrayals of the human condition. It was the end of October, and it was snowing in Baltimore. This led to delays in traffic, and my plan to arrive well before the start of the film was falling apart. Traffic slowed to a trickle, and I was in a frazzled state when I parked my car outside the theater. To make matters worse, as I stepped out, I landed my foot deep in an icy puddle. I made my way through the snow, soaked and upset, into the theater. I had hoped it would be relatively empty, but it was packed, of course. The film was already 15 minutes in. I did not even glance at the screen, scrambling around until I found an empty seat. I climbed over half a row of people and settled in, gloomily subdued, my heart rate and breathing accelerated by all the preceding events. I looked up at the screen, and there was a woman seated by the window, staring languidly outside as she prepared her potatoes. There was no dialogue, but a melancholy musical score drifted elegantly over the scene. I sat with her, shared her view, with no further action taking place for a considerable time. Abandoning the hyperkinetic state I was in and finding myself in the midst of such contemplative stillness was a contrast I did not expect. I surrendered to the experience. The chaos of the outside world could wait. Now was my time to stop, to listen, to take in.

This anecdote has stuck with me as an example of what psychotherapy can offer. Patients enter our consulting rooms bearing the burden of life's relentless assaults on their peace of mind. We invite them to slow down and allow thought to emerge without being rushed by the familiar worldly pressures that mercilessly demand concrete results in minimal time frames. We attempt to join our patients in this stillness, allowing the richness of their internal worlds to be expressed.

Each patient has a unique subjectivity informed by childhood experiences, by hopes realized and dashed, by moments of joy and bitter disappointment, and by the weight of accumulating losses that inevitably accompany the passage of time. A patient's subjective experience of the provider (what is termed *transference*), including expectations about how the latter will think and behave, is influenced by how life events have shaped the patient's psyche. The converse is true as well. As patients speak to us, our *own* minds, informed by our own preconceptions, life histories, and linguistic and cultural lenses, filter what we hear into something intelligible and digestible to *us*. As their trajectories intersect with ours in the clinical encounter, we try to find a common language despite the endless differences between the subjects in the room.

On what level does this communication happen? No matter how much we may summon our training, our white coats, our diagnostic manuals and criteria, our medications, and our treatment algorithms, we are fundamentally relating to our patients as one human to another. While we need the tools listed to help guide aspects of treatment, it is through the cultivation of a psychodynamic thought process that we can deepen and enrich our understanding of a patient's struggles and life story. Such thinking implicates *us* as well, as active participants in a dyad seeking to identify the bedrock linking our common humanity despite any objective differences. Dynamic therapy is unique in that it can sometimes feel as though there are *two* patients in the room, as we open ourselves up to our own emotional responses to patients. Such openness to the unexpected can lead us down scary roads. As Wilfred Bion stated, "In every consulting room there ought to be two rather frightened people: the patient and the psycho-analyst" (Bion 1990, p. 5). We use *countertransference*—our own subjective responses to patients—as a diagnostic tool that helps us understand them better. We take our minds home with us, we mull, we worry, we let their conflicts keep us up at night. We struggle with them to make sense of their internal worlds. Helping them is an imperfect art but an art all the same.

We must always be open to learning something new from every patient encounter, even if it is with someone we have seen for years. When I teach psychodynamic formulation (i.e., how to connect present life struggles with a patient's developmental history), I liken the process of writing a formulation to creating a mandala. We put a great deal of thought and care into how we think about patients; we build gorgeously eloquent verbal edifices paying tribute to our holistic understanding of where our patients came from and where they are now. Yet we need to be ready to dismantle these constructs entirely and let go of our illusion of any permanence in our understanding. As we maintain this soft, flexible stance toward what we hear in therapy, without pathologizing what we are told or funneling it through lists of criteria, patients may also adopt such a model, giving *themselves* permission to reflect on their own minds in more nuanced and complex ways. This softening of ingrained, rigid conceptualizations of themselves allows our patients to learn from experience, imbuing their lives with a renewed sense of wonder and spontaneity. Life is infinite in its possibilities and varieties. As we embark on the quest of accessing our patients' inner worlds, we are privileged to be the ones to whom the inexpressible is finally uttered. We are the quiet presence offering a space for contemplation, a nonjudgmental approach to whatever our patients have to say, and a respite from the frenzy of an unrelenting world that seems increasingly devoid of empathy.

It is not uncommon in this accelerated profession to short-circuit more discerning thinking, robbing patients of their right to subjective richness. Terms like *psychopath*, *crazy*, *malingerer*, and much worse are thrown around like verbal shrapnel, without compunction or second thought. The need for a measured, careful, empathic approach is more pressing than ever. As the relevance of damaging biases has gained renewed focus, we are attempting to take steps toward a more self-critical stance, but there is much work to be done. Patients come to us for healing, and many times they are met with intolerance, with staff who split them off as beyond hope and not worth their time. Many times, the patients who are treated the worst are those who have had the most challenges throughout life; unknowingly, we may be recapitulating traumatic experiences and solidifying the patients' impressions that such dispiriting outcomes are the only possible ones when their emotional world is laid bare.

Focus and Intended Audience

This book is my attempt to emphasize the continued importance of psychodynamic thought in contemporary psychotherapy education. I work in an academic setting and have always held that psychoanalysis belongs in universities. It needs to be part of the discussion, as opposed to split off and kept in some capsule away from the mainstream of training programs. Educators of the next generation of mental health providers need to be aware of how transference and countertransference dynamics critically inform how we view, discuss, interact with, and treat our patients. With this in mind, this book presents the principles of psychodynamic psychotherapy from a clinician-educator's perspective. Knowing well that a career as a psychotherapist or psychoanalyst may not be of particular interest to many trainees, I have tried to adopt an experience-near approach in presenting the material. Most of the discussion pertains to conducting psychotherapy sessions in an office, but I also present some examples from acute levels of care, illustrating how the principles being discussed transcend settings. Although I have completed psychoanalytic training and maintained active engagement with dynamic therapy and psychoanalysis, I have also worked for years in the psychiatric emergency department, and this has helped me realize that thinking dynamically about patients outside traditional therapy settings is not only useful but quite crucial.

My approach has been informed by years of teaching psychodynamic theory and practice, developing curricula, and maintaining engagement with the psychoanalytic and residency education communities. Importantly, fostering a concurrent grounding in developments in the neurosciences has helped me find ways of reconciling concepts from psychological and biological fields. Findings in neurobiology have advanced our understanding of child development (including attachment paradigms), biomarkers correlating with diagnosed psychiatric conditions, and the therapeutic action of psychotherapy. Unexpectedly, my engagement with biological theories has consolidated the relevance and applicability of object relations theory. It is a perspective that finds a strong resonance with the neurobiological underpinnings of development. Namely, neuroscientific models have posited that environmental effects (including interactions with early figures) are encoded during sensitive periods of childhood, locking in a cognitive and affective "map" that consolidates an individual's sense of self and others. Indeed, it is biologically cumbersome to reroute these early maps, given how important quick and efficient encoding is for the developing brain. As such, self-other interactions, along with their emotional quality, become templates for how relationships will operate in later life. This aligns with the notion of how one develops models of object relationships that become internalized (see "Defining Object Relations" below). The neuroscientific aspects of object relations will be developed at length in Chapter 10 ("A Neuroscientific Perspective on Object Relations").

Additionally, the *ubiquity* of object relationships makes this psychodynamic model particularly compelling because it is relevant to *every* patient encounter, in *any* setting. As we pay attention to the aliveness of the relationship in the room, we notice how patients may be experiencing us, as well as what our *own* emotional reactions to them may be. (Such reactions can be very strong indeed). In creating a space for such attentiveness to be cultivated, we learn about a patient's history in vivid ways. We might notice ourselves being treated like figures from our patients' past (we might even *feel* some of the emotions being attributed to us), viewed as we are through the lens of their previous experiences, which generate expectations and particular forms of relating to us. From this vantage point, the basic unit of understanding in a clinical encounter is the *object relationship*.

The relevance of the object relations model from clinical and biological perspectives uniquely positions it to help further psychodynamic education in training programs for mental health professionals. This backdrop informs the object relations lens, which is the guiding orientation of the book. I have, when it was necessary to do so, brought in concepts from other schools of psychoanalytic thought to help consolidate certain discussion points.

With regard to the intended audience, this book is for learners as well as educators. By *learners*, I mean anyone acquiring an education about psychodynamic psychotherapy with the intention of applying it to clinical or academic work. This may include graduate or postgraduate students across mental health disciplines, psychoanalytic candidates, and those who have an established practice and wish to familiarize themselves with an object relations perspective.

Although my work has been geared mainly toward psychiatric residents, I have constructed this book with a much broader audience in mind. Irrespective of background, dynamic principles can greatly enrich our appreciation of many facets of human expression.

Defining Object Relations

> [T]here is always an object relationship in the consulting room and [...] our first task is to be aware of the active nature of this relationship.
>
> Betty Joseph (1988, p. 631)

There are as many forms of doing psychotherapy as there are psychotherapists. After all, the subjectivity of the provider is brought into the room and becomes *part* of the technical approach. Sigmund Freud had his own views on countertransference, positing at one point that it was something to be "overcome" by the provider (Freud 1910/1955), allowing for a more "objective" appraisal of what a patient was expressing. However, we have come to appreciate that the therapist's countertransference is not only inevitable but also *welcome* and *necessary* for the work to be done.[1] While some psychoanalytic schools may place emphasis on reconstructions of the "how" and "when" particular events might have shaped an individual's emotional and behavioral trajectories in life, there is always the danger of screen memories and affective distortions to any objective description of fact, making the historical veracity of past accounts at best an approximation.

An object relations approach offers an attractive alternative to such reconstructions: the "here and now" dimension of the psychotherapeutic dyad. In other words, the question that is always to be asked is: "What is taking place in the room at this time between my patient and me?" We may represent someone different to a given patient at different times, sometimes from *one moment to the next* within a single session. The mind is not stagnant, and we seek to make contact with something perpetually in motion, as patients view us through the lens of their internal object worlds. In what follows I provide brief, working definitions of some key terms that I will return to throughout the book.

External Objects, Splitting, and Projection

The term *object* can generate some degree of confusion in terms of meaning and clinical applicability.[2] Simply stated, we can think of an *external object* as a physical, real human with whom one interacts. The earliest objects in one's life will have an instrumental role in shaping one's understanding not only of the external environment but also of one's internal state. Objects in the child's life will be assigned particular qualities depending on the nature of the interactions. Critically, a child may project something of the self's own *internal* state onto the object, now viewed not objectively but in a way tinged by fantasy.[3,4]

---

[1] Throughout the book, when "Freud" is referenced, it is to be inferred that Sigmund Freud is the author in question, unless otherwise specified.

[2] Freud used the word *object* in different ways. In "Instincts and Their Vicissitudes" (Freud 1915/1955), he outlined how the expression of drive or libido occurs through a source, aim, and object; he defined an object as "the thing in regard to which or through which the instinct is able to achieve its aim" (p. 122). In "On Narcissism" (Freud 1914/1955), in discussing how libido is cathected, he distinguished between ego-libido (love toward self) and object-libido (love toward the other); he stated, "The highest phase of development of which object-libido is capable is seen in the state of being in love, when the subject seems to give up his own personality in favour of an object-cathexis" (Freud 1914/1955, p. 76). Of note, I am defining *cathexis* as the psychic energy that is invested in the individual's mental representation of an object, thought, desire, or feeling.

In accordance with developmentally determined abilities, the infant will interact with external objects in partial ways, through the function they are (or are not) serving at a given time. A child who is feeling warm, satiated, and appeased may assign the power to generate such a state to an external object. This object—experienced according to the function or role it serves, with no greater dimensionality to it beyond bearing responsibility for the child's internal state—will be an *all-good, part-object* for this child.[5] It is this all-good object that gives the child that feeling of having a belly full of warm, good stuff, allowing for such contented bliss. Similarly, a child in distress (e.g., cold, wet, hungry) may assign the responsibility for this distress to an *all-bad, part-object*, one felt to be actively inflicting this terrible state onto the child. (Notably, such feelings will be experienced not as the "absence of the good object," but rather as though there were an evil, harmful object *causing* discomfort, tugging away at the child's tummy and generating the uncomfortable wetness and cold.)

In this primitive mode of patterning the environment, the "bad" and the "good" experiences are kept separate, a separation referred to as *splitting*. As the child attributes something of the self to the object (e.g., a bad internal feeling), we see how something is split off from inside the child and projected out. This *projection* will influence how the child experiences external objects, now assigned something of the child's as though it were the object's.

Internal Objects

The interactions a child has with external objects will lead to internalized mental and emotional representations of the objects. These representations

---

[3] The ubiquity of fantasy in tingeing how individuals perceive objects was emphasized by Susan Isaacs (1948). Indeed, it could be argued an external object is never viewed objectively because our emotional and cognitive state in any given moment influences how the object is being experienced.

[4] The reader will note a difference in spelling of the word *fantasy*. Isaacs (1948) recommended the spelling "phantasy" for unconscious phenomena (she referred to phantasy as "the mental corollary, the psychic representative, of instinct" [p. 81] and "fantasy" for "conscious day-dreams, fictions, and so on" [p. 80]). Such distinctions have been challenged because indeed "it is often difficult to be sure whether a patient's phantasy is unconscious, tacitly conscious or fully conscious" (Spillius et al. 2011, p. 5). A number of British analysts use *phantasy* to refer to both conscious and unconscious phenomena. In this book, with the exception of direct quotes, I have adopted the "fantasy" spelling, without distinguishing between conscious and unconscious content.

[5] The earliest prototype of this part-object relationship has been characterized as a nursing baby at the breast.

can be termed *internal objects* and serve structuring functions for the developing child's mind. The internalized good object (derived from interactions that prove satisfying and comforting) will pattern the existence of a force in the world that provides the child with a life-affirming, soothing, and integrating experience, the internalization of which gives the child something within the self to draw from when faced with anxiety and needing to self-soothe. Conversely, the internalized bad object (derived from situations leading to *unresolved* distress) is the pull toward disintegration, pain, and confusion. The child will access these internal objects when interacting with others in the future, creating (through projection) expectancies surrounding the state of mind and intention of others based on early templates.

With a predominance of "good" over "bad" experiences, a basic sense of safety will be established. As the child interacts with sensitive caregivers capable of attuning to the child's inner experience and providing a soothing response, what will be progressively internalized is that one's internal state can be safely processed. The child will thus not feel the need to project as much into the object when feeling distress because this uncomfortable feeling has been shown to be manageable as opposed to catastrophic. (This also leads to the child's being able to experience negative or aggressive feelings as parts of the self, as opposed to being attributed to the doings of an all-bad object.) Similarly, when feeling good, the child will not necessarily assign responsibility to an external object but rather may internalize the ability to self-soothe, as modeled by caregivers. As this process unfolds, the child is able to experience both self and objects with greater dimensionality, lessening splitting and projection. An understanding emerges that the "separate" good and bad part-objects were actually aspects of the *same* object. Appreciating objects with this level of nuance is to view them as *whole objects*. As detailed earlier, splitting entails severing awareness of something within the self in order to project it into the object; in other words, *splitting of the object also necessitates a splitting of the self*. As the child progresses to whole-object relating, this also allows for greater understanding of one's *own* traits, now viewed as belonging to the self as opposed to needing to be projected out. In other words, it can be highly integrating for a child to experience moments of attunement with caregivers.[6]

As Elizabeth Bott Spillius and colleagues (2011, p. 40) stated,

> The introjection of and identification with a stable good object is crucial to the ego's capacity to cohere and integrate experience. Damaged or dead in-

---

[6] Melanie Klein (1957/1975) stated, "An infant who has securely established the good object can also find compensations for loss and deprivation in adult life" (p. 204).

ternal objects cause enormous anxiety and can lead to personality disintegration, whereas objects felt to be in a good state promote confidence and well-being.

Over the life course, new experiences with external objects lead to an updating of one's internal objects, which may acquire new features and enrich the individual's sense of self and of the world. Indeed, such an updating occurs in the developing child (e.g., in the transition from part- to whole-object relating). It is also part of the therapeutic action in treatment, as patients present with conflicts and symptoms that may stem from harsher internal objects. Through patients' work with the new object of the therapist, if the latter is able to provide a space for reflection and processing, what becomes internalized is not a carbon copy of previously known objects (though this may happen in short-lived, unproductive treatments) but rather a more flexible, understanding, and supportive object that patients will carry with them as part of their (now modified) internal worlds. Such an updating will be important in softening one's expectations of self and (in some cases) lessening the need to be punished when such expectations are not met (see the discussion of the superego in Chapter 8, "The Oedipal Situation [Exclusion and Rivalry]: Theory").

Projective Identification

Progressing from part-object to whole-object relating hinges, as mentioned, on caregiver attunement to the child's internal state, providing the child with the feeling of having been understood, with a concomitant lessening of inner discomfort.

At the beginning of this process, the distressed child's discomfort is communicated to the caregiver, with the child perhaps even projecting onto the latter the "all-bad" traits of an object *causing* the child to feel so distraught. If the object "takes on" the projection—not turning away from the distressed child but rather leaning into the situation, "owning" the child's distress in an attempt to join the child in feeling it and to help relieve it—a two-person dynamic is active, turning one person's distress into a joint, dyadic processing. This is an example of *projective identification.*[7] Importantly, the object's participation is essential for this defense to lead to healthy outcomes. Projective identification is, fundamentally, a form of communication. A child does not have words to express inner feelings and thoughts; thus the child's gestures

---

[7] Readers are referred to the paper by Feldman (1992) titled "Splitting and Projective Identification" for a useful clinical example differentiating projection from projective identification.

and sounds require a caregiver presence beyond ordinary language, a desire to know and to provide comfort, a wish to actually be drawn into the child's experience in order to assist with making sense of the child's inner world. It is profoundly reassuring for both parties when such primitive communication takes place, and indeed it has been said that projective identification is the basis for empathy. If we think about the above-mentioned example of a caregiver successfully attuning to and relieving the child's distress, a situation in which the caregiver could have been experienced as a bad object (e.g., had there been dyadic misattunement) was transformed, through projective identification, into a good-object experience. Such an exchange is internalized by the child, whose internal object world will be updated, (re)affirming the presence of the internal good object.

In his seminal paper on projective identification, Thomas Ogden spoke of three stages in this defense: 1) "the fantasy of projecting a part of oneself into another person and of that part taking over the person from within"; 2) "pressure exerted via the interpersonal interaction such that the 'recipient' of the projection experiences pressure to think, feel, and behave in a manner congruent with the projection"; and 3) the projector's reinternalizing of "the projected feelings, after being 'psychologically processed' by the recipient" (Ogden 1979, p. 358). (This third step is, of course, what caregivers—as well as therapists treating patients—wish to achieve.)

The containing function of the caregivers allows them to be present for and attuned to their children, responding "in a manner that makes the infant feel it is receiving its frightened personality back again, but in a form that it can tolerate" (Bion 1962b, p. 308). The caregiver will show evidence of having been affected by the baby's state but not so much that it causes undue distress beyond the caregiver's abilities to both cope and be present for the child. The latter thus will experience the event as the caregiver having come into contact with something terrible and tolerating it. This models a capacity to hold onto these projected bits and process them and detoxify them, and over time this will aid the child in reducing projective defenses and in tolerating these feelings that felt so overwhelming before. It is this active process of taking in the baby's projections and metabolizing them into something that can be fed back in a manageable way that is the essence of the *container* function modeled by the caregiver, as described by Bion (1962a).[8]

As will be discussed in Chapter 6 ("Developing a Sense of Self: Theory") and Chapter 7 ("Developing a Sense of Self: Clinical"), a lack of containing experiences (e.g., caused by misattuned or abusive caregivers) may interfere

---

[8] Particularly Chapters 27 and 28.

with the child's development of an integrated sense of self and progression to whole-object relating. Rather, there may be a persistence of part-object relating, with a predominance of splitting and strong projective defenses, restricting the child's understanding of self and others to rigid templates. An internal world occupied by harsher objects may result, generating uncertainty, fear, and emotional-cognitive immobility at the expense of curiosity and psychic growth. Returning to the earlier example of the distressed child and the caregiver, let us imagine a scenario in which the latter was overwhelmed by the child's incessant crying and fussiness, perhaps yelling at the child or walking away in a state of agitation. Indeed, we can think of this as the caregiver taking on those bad object traits but being unable to reach the third stage described by Ogden, in which the experience can be transformed into something more integrating and growth-promoting for the child. This is also an instance of projective identification, wherein the caregiver identified with (in effect, *became*) the bad object. The child's unprocessed distress may be *worsened* by the "confirmation" of an external object who is unable to help the child feel better. Rather, the caregiver conforms to the projected role of an object that indeed forces the child to deal with this unbearable distress alone; in some ways, it becomes a situation in which the caregiver really may appear to be *inflicting* these terrible feelings on the child. It is this type of object that will be introjected into the child's internal world, potentially serving as a point of reference as to how these situations will unfold the next time the child feels similarly distraught.

Projective identification will remain at the center of how we interact with others. If more primitive forms persist, projective identification will be used in the service of ridding oneself of something unwanted, relating to others as mindless receptacles for traits with which one wishes to disidentify (I will elaborate on this shortly). This may lead to poor boundaries and impoverishment of the sense of self, including where the self ends and the other begins (because the latter is "in possession of" this projected bit). For instance, in borderline personality disorder (BPD), splitting and projective identification are resorted to frequently; patients with BPD may view others as all good, projecting their liveliness and sense of self into the other, which may factor into the feelings of emptiness and terror of being abandoned that can accompany this condition. If the idealized other leaves, it may feel as though the patient with BPD is left with a gaping psychic hole because the all-good person, the one supposedly "holding the patient together," has been torn away, with no sturdy sense of an individuated self remaining. (This underlines the idea that an all-good object can quickly become all bad, accounting for rapid shifts in how others are perceived, especially if they fail to conform to a particular part-object configuration.) We can compare this in a sense to the way in which the baby experiences the caregiver as all-giving and integrating; because of its very nature, the caregiver-object in effect contains not only all-good abilities but potentially all-bad qualities as well. If the caregiver were to leave, this would in effect deprive the baby of a presence believed to be necessary for survival. Thus, embedded within an idealized object is the potential for destructiveness, lending credence to the notion that the flip-side of an idealized object is a persecutory object. To quote Klein (1957/1975), "Infants whose capacity for love is strong feel less need for idealization than those in whom destructive impulses and persecutory anxiety are paramount. Excessive idealization denotes that persecution is the main driving force" (pp. 192–193).

In more mature forms, projective identification is used in the service of empathizing with others. In whole-object relating, an individual who is attempting to process an internal experience may try to convey to an object a sense of what is being struggled with. In effect, the mind of the other is recruited to try to make sense of one's internal state. If I wish to have someone understand what I am feeling, I will try to evoke an image, explanation, or emotional state that relays what is on my mind. If I succeed, my situation will be sensed by the object, whose thinking apparatus will be recruited to help me process it and assign meaning. If the object is successful, I will be able to take back in my projection, in a metabolized state, and expand my self-awareness and self-understanding. Critically, at no point did I *disown* this internal trait and view it as "belonging" to the other; rather, I "knew it was mine" and wished to update my understanding of myself with the assistance of a trusted other's thought process.

Alternatively, when one is grappling with an internal state one does *not* wish to view as one's own (perhaps because it was not processed, metabolized, and assigned meaning by a caregiver earlier in life, making it difficult for the child to assimilate the trait as one's own), projective identification serves a much more forceful purpose. Such a trait or internal state will be split off and projected into the object, who will then be viewed as *possessing* it. However, unlike the mature form described before, the objective is *not* to reclaim the trait after the object's metabolizing process makes it more palatable. Rather, the object is there to serve as a receptacle for something unwanted located within the projector. This depletes the latter of one's completeness while reducing the object to a two-dimensional construct viewed through the lens of the projected trait. Thus, the object can only serve a role—to hold onto the projection, in effect serving as a part-object. Given the inability to view the trait as part of the self, efforts will mount to force the object to identify with the projection. For instance, if an individual grew up with caregivers who ridiculed the child anytime the latter displayed any sign of incompetence, this trait will continue to signal danger in the person's mind because it is equated with loss of caregiver attention, esteem, and love. Thus, locating "incompetence" in others may serve to rid the self of such a noxious trait. The individual may be quite attuned to signs of incompetence in other people and "jump on" any opportunity to point out their failures. If the other person indeed "feels" incompetent, the projector will feel a sense of relief because this will be confirmation that incompetence is *not* a part of the self but rather a problem *other* people have to deal with. Perceptions of others thus will be strongly biased, given one's unease in viewing the self in possession of certain problematic characteristics. To revisit one's take would potentially invite anxiety and an unbearable sense of groundlessness because the terrible situation with the mocking caregiver would be psychically revisited (on a conscious and/or unconscious level). Thus, selective attention to realities that confirm one's two-dimensional view will be fostered, while those that challenge this perspective will be ignored (akin to "confirmation bias"). As James Fosshage (2004) stated, "Experience of the world that is discrepant with expectancies is disruptive and challenges current views of reality. These disruptions jeopardize self-cohesion, self-regulation and the capacity to negotiate" (p. 54).

When interacting with others, we are all influenced by our individual internal object organizations, no matter how much training and self-reflection we might have undertaken. As therapists, we wish to be open to our patients without being overly burdened by *our own* preconceptions or by too much theory. Of course, we bring our own internal worlds into clinical encounters, and there is no way of eliminating the influence of our internal objects. Rather, we cultivate a sensitivity to our countertransference in ways that (hopefully) further our sense of how we are being perceived by patients at given moments. However, there are times when our own conflicts and introjects can overly organize our thinking and interventions. We may even say something clumsy or hostile that creates awkwardness in a session. This is unavoidable given the nature of the work. However, it need not be viewed as detrimental; rather, it can be viewed as something to be learned from, something enacted and survived by the dyad, to be processed in subsequent sessions. As I will discuss in Chapter 2 ("Starting Psychotherapy Supervision"), we can enhance our awareness of the contributions of our own internal object worlds through personal treatment and processing material with our supervisors and colleagues.

Just as we need to be careful not to let our subjectivity cloud our perception of patients, we also need to be judicious in how theory is utilized. In my mind, theory is crucial, yet it is ancillary and always to be used in the service of facilitating our receptiveness to the individual in front of us, as opposed to serving as a substitute for learning about the new and rich universe contained in every patient we see. If we overly organize patients' material through theorizing channels, it becomes less about the person we are seeing and more about us funneling what we are hearing to accord with what we already know. The real person with whom we are interacting is essentially lost, and we are basically left conversing with our own minds. Theory is important, but we need to be able to hold onto it softly and let it go to be fully present during sessions.

The Object Relations Lens

Given this exposition of relevant concepts, I will now outline, in simplified form, how one might construct an "object relations lens" that can be referred to in the clinical encounter, reflecting the principles that will be greatly expanded upon over the course of this work.[9]

- Every patient has a subjectivity, which is always present in the clinical encounter.
- Patients experience and interact with the therapist in accordance with their internalized relationship templates.
- The internal object world of the *therapist* will factor into how the patient is perceived and responded to.
- All clinical encounters are influenced by how the respective internal object worlds of therapist and patient interact.

Structure of the Book

I have conceptualized this work as composed of two main sections:

Chapters 2 through 5 present practical aspects of getting started with patients in psychotherapy. In Chapter 2, I underline the importance of psychotherapy supervision and provide some suggestions as to how it may be productively used. In the subsequent three chapters, I discuss the importance of the therapeutic frame, the meaning of the therapist's interventions, the uses and limitations of silence, and how to think of the matter of "process" versus "content" when listening to patients' associations. All of these technical aspects are considered vis-à-vis the active object relationship in the room: the patient-therapist dyad. Because many trainees may be starting therapy

---

[9] Although I draw primarily from the works of Melanie Klein, Donald Winnicott, Wilfred Bion, and the modern Kleinians, it must be acknowledged that there are several theorists whose contributions have been invaluable to the evolution of object relations theory and practice. These include Ronald Fairbairn, Harry Guntrip, Michael Balint, and Otto Kernberg. Because of space constraints, I have not been able to do justice to the scope and breadth of their work within this volume.

with a minimum of theoretical grounding, I have constructed these chapters to address common, practical dimensions of engaging with patients, without being weighed down by too much theoretical exposition (beyond what has been provided as foundational knowledge in this introduction). Indeed, in many ways, this matches the trajectory of some training programs, because the acquisition of theory takes place along the academic year in tandem with ongoing clinical work.

Chapters 6 through 10 present more advanced concepts from object relations theory. Namely, Chapters 6 and 7 discuss developmental considerations from roughly the first 3 years of life, when more dyadic forms of relating predominate. I expand primarily on the theories of Donald Winnicott, Melanie Klein, and Wilfred Bion in discussing how a sense of self is fostered during these years, noting the critical role of early objects in the child's world in consolidating selfhood. Chapters 8 and 9 discuss the subsequent period in development, aligned with the Oedipal situation and the child's negotiation of triadic relationships. My theoretical basis in these two chapters derives largely from the works of Klein and Margaret Mahler. Early life is thus divided into dyadic and triadic stages. Readers will note that each of these sections has two chapters dedicated to them. For each stage, I have chosen to present a theoretical chapter first followed by a more clinically oriented one. In the clinical chapters, I illustrate how these early life psychic modes of functioning can continue to present in adult life, including how we may notice them in clinical encounters. Critically, these chapters highlight how an individual may *oscillate* between these two modes of functioning (i.e., between the dyadic mode [aligned with the paranoid-schizoid position] and the triadic mode [aligned with the depressive position]). Thus, Chapters 6 through 9 together provide a more nuanced appreciation of how this object relations lens can be implemented in therapy (and, to some extent, in acute care settings, as I will illustrate).

The technical approach espoused in this book is twofold and sequential: 1) to cultivate the space to observe and experience the object relationship in the room (largely the focus described in Chapters 2 through 5) and 2) to deepen our thinking about this relationship in light of the patient's early development (elaborated in Chapters 6 through 9). As suggested by the opening quote in this book, it is important to sustain something grounded and thinking within ourselves even when faced with a flurry of outside activity. This is very relevant for the clinical encounters, which may evoke powerful emotional reactions in both members of the dyad. The ability to reach our patients and serve as healing objects hinges on our capacity to maintain a grounded presence, receptive to their internal worlds yet not being pulled into harmful reenactments that recapitulate traumatic templates. These technical precepts can help providers foster this attentive and flexible presence for patients, whether in psychotherapy or in other clinical settings.[10]

Chapter 10 presents a neuroscientific understanding of object relations. It is arguably the most technical chapter in the book, but I have tried to tie in the neurobiological descriptions with the psychodynamic terminology presented previously, to aid with assimilation.

Chapter 11 explores the many facets of termination, focusing primarily on treatments that are ending because of the time-limited nature of training programs, as opposed to reflecting on when a particular patient is deemed ready to terminate because of clinical improvement (a subject that is beyond the scope of this book, though references are provided for interested readers).

A Note on Language

In this book, I refer to *trainees* and *residents* somewhat interchangeably. I believe these precepts apply broadly within and beyond the medical field, but because many of my teaching experiences are with psychiatry residents, at times this term makes its appearance even though the concepts being discussed are not limited to the work of residency. I have tried to use the term *trainee* when positing more general principles and clinical examples and *resident* when discussing specific examples from my own teaching experience.

When presenting process material from clinical sessions, I use the letter *T* to refer to myself or the provider in question (therapist) and the letter *P* to refer to the patient. Throughout the book, with respect to nonbinary appellations, I have elected, when speaking of general principles, to use the pronoun *they* when referring to individuals, which is why readers may observe the use of the plural *patients* at several points. Notably, the pronoun *they* may at times also be used when referring to a singular individual (including children). (Such use has garnered increasing acceptance in both colloquial and academic realms; see Baron 2018.)

Because patient confidentiality is of capital importance in this profession, all case vignettes derived from clinical encounters have been extensively modified and disguised to preserve anonymity. Some of the vignettes have

---

[10] There are therapeutic modalities in which the transference-countertransference dynamic is the primary guide to the therapist's interpretations. This can be handled beautifully in sessions; the modern Kleinian school exemplifies such an approach. The lens advocated by this book aligns with a similar mode of thinking about patients and clinical encounters; however, it should be reiterated that this work is not a primer on systematic transference interpretations. Such a technique is well beyond the scope of this book (and anathema to making these concepts more accessible to early learners).

been constructed de novo to illustrate salient points pertaining to the material being discussed.

KEY POINTS

- The object relations model provides us with a framework to understand how early life shapes one's "working models" of interactions between self and others. These models will be carried forward and relived in later relationships.

- The term *object* can denote a person with whom one has interacted (external object) and an internalized representation of this person (internal object), the latter carrying one's cognitive and visceral memories of how this object was experienced.

- Through the defense of projective identification, internal representations of early objects can be "pushed onto others," who will then be seen through the lens of projection, creating the expectation that the "new" external object will behave like the "old" one.

- During any given interaction between two people, each will be viewing the other through the lens of the respective internal object worlds.

- The object relations lens is of the utmost clinical relevance because *every* patient we encounter will have a developmental history and an internal object world that will shape how we are viewed. By embracing the richness of our patients' subjective experiences and observing the dynamics of our interactions, we can understand the relationship models that have been consolidated, in ways that may be difficult to express in words.

References

Baron D: A brief history of singular "they" (blog). Oxford English Dictionary 2018. Available at: https://public.oed.com/blog/a-brief-history-of-singular-they/#. Accessed May 12, 2021.

Bion W: Learning From Experience. London, Karnac, 1962a

Bion WR: The psycho-analytic study of thinking: a theory of thinking. Int J Psychoanal 43:306–310, 1962b 13968380

Bion W: Brazilian Lectures: 1973, São Paulo; 1974, Rio de Janeiro/São Paulo. Oxon, UK, Routledge, 1990

Feldman M: Splitting and projective identification. New Library of Psychoanalysis 14:74–88, 1992

Fosshage JL: The explicit and implicit dance in psychoanalytic change. J Anal Psychol 49(1):49–65, 2004 14720229

Freud S: The future prospects of psycho-analytic therapy (1910), in The Standard Edition of the Complete Psychological Works of Sigmund Freud, Vol 11. Translated and edited by Strachey J. London, Hogarth Press, 1955, pp 139–152

Freud S: On narcissism (1914), in The Standard Edition of the Complete Psychological Works of Sigmund Freud, Vol 14. Translated and edited by Strachey J. London, Hogarth Press, 1955, pp 67–102

Freud S: Instincts and their vicissitudes (1915), in The Standard Edition of the Complete Psychological Works of Sigmund Freud, Vol 14. Translated and edited by Strachey J. London, Hogarth Press, 1955, pp 109–140

Isaacs S: The nature and function of phantasy. Int J Psychoanal 29:73–97, 1948

Joseph B: Object relations in clinical practice. Psychoanal Q 57(4):626–642, 1988 3212106

Juniper A: Wabi Sabi: The Japanese Art of Impermanence. North Clarendon, VT, Tuttle Publishing, 2003

Klein M: Envy and gratitude (1957), in Envy and Gratitude and Other Works 1946–1963. Edited by Khan M. London, Hogarth Press, 1975, pp 176–235

Ogden TH: On projective identification. Int J Psychoanal 60 (Pt 3):357–373, 1979 533737

Spillius EB, Milton J, Garvey P, et al: The New Dictionary of Kleinian Thought. New York, Routledge, 2011

Starting Psychotherapy Supervision

Whatever you become, teacher, scholar, or musician, have respect for the "meaning," but do not imagine that it can be taught.

Hermann Hesse (1943/2012, p. 122)

BEFORE EMBARKING on a discussion of the practical aspects of psychotherapy, I am going to reflect on the important role of supervision in one's development as a therapist, particularly when one is first engaging in this type of clinical work.

The Difficult Adjustment

Starting therapy with patients can be overwhelming and anxiety provoking, as well as an adjustment from a very different way of thinking about and working with patients. In many psychiatry residency programs, for instance, the outpatient year is preceded by a year or two of managing patients in more acute settings (e.g., inpatient units, consultation services, psychiatric emergency department). During these rotations, time spent with patients may be limited and diagnostically oriented, prioritizing a working assessment and treatment plan. This guides the team's thinking over the course of the hospital stay, with some allowance for reconceptualization as new data are gathered and the patient is seen once or twice daily until discharge. However, providers may find themselves holding to initial diagnostic impressions and limiting the scope of subsequent interviews, focusing on how the presenting symptoms have changed (or not) in response to interventions—not that this approach is problematic in any way, because we need to be sure we are appropriately addressing symptoms that suggest specific diagnoses. Indeed, this is probably the *necessary* focus when there are more acute concerns, when safety and stabilization are the priorities. It can feel very grounding to have a working diagnosis and concrete treatment plan, as well as a set list of questions to monitor progress. On inpatient units, patients are there overnight, and we are essentially assured they will be there in the morning when we arrive for work.

It is a momentous shift when residents move from these settings into the outpatient world, where the guardrails go away. Although there may still be some similarities in "medication management" sessions or in more manualized forms of therapy, it is a very different framework when long-term psychodynamic therapy is initiated. Our questionnaires will only take us so far before we are in open waters, without a map to give us a sense of direction. We no longer know where we will be taken. When sessions end, patients go home. We hope they will be back next time, but there is always the possibility they will not be, an uncertainty that may cause us to second-guess ourselves and catastrophize about what we did wrong if a patient is late or is a no-show for the following session. Also, the more we learn about our patients in therapy, the less useful diagnoses become. We start to appreciate how limiting such constructs are in encompassing a subjectivity that is greater than any explanatory terms we may assign to it, much like characters in a play who are much more complex and alive than the scripted lines they read would suggest. When we abandon our much-valued control, it can feel like the floor is being taken out from under us.

I remember my own transition. After 12 months of inpatient and emergency department work, I started my outpatient year thinking I knew everything. After 1 year of working with patients in psychotherapy, I told my supervisor, "I think I'm a worse therapist at the end of this year than I was at the beginning." His response surprised me: "I'm so glad to hear you say that." In retrospect, I had been blinded by the omniscience of a different mode of working, in which we assume we *know* what is happening with the patient and what needs to be done. All this is quickly undone when we create the opportunity for something new to find its way in.

Starting therapy work with patients is like jumping into cold water: there is no easy way of doing it, and no amount of inching will necessarily make it easier. Even if someone has great interest in therapy and has read extensively on the topic, it is an entirely unique experience sitting in front of one's patients and attempting to find their psychic knots and learn how they came to be tied. None of the psychiatric literature, after all, will have addressed what is happening in the immediacy of this new setting, with *this* therapist and *this* patient engaging in *this* session. Sessions are always uncharted waters, even if we have vast theoretical grounding.

Many who gravitate toward the mental health field consider themselves good listeners and are interested in hearing people's stories. Indeed, this is a common self-description mentioned by medical students who are applying to psychiatry residency programs. Yet understanding what makes every individual unique and complex is an endless quest. Aspiring psychotherapists need guidance on how to engage in this art form of helping people through conversation. No two internal worlds are alike, and even patients with the same diagnosis and reported symptoms have entirely distinct subjectivities and life trajectories.

One of the key tools to help hone the skills of trainees is *psychotherapy supervision*, which typically occurs in a weekly, one-to-one format. Supervision may represent the trainee's first formal introduction to the world of psychodynamic thought. The supervisor's technical approach and theoretical orientation, as well as how the supervisory hour is structured, will be key aspects of what a trainee takes away from the experience and is able to apply to patient care. It is the job of the supervisor to serve as a supportive figure for the trainee, to help process what is happening in the sessions, and to provide guidance when treatment impasses or empathic ruptures occur. Therapists many times get pulled into the intensity of patients' inner worlds, leading to reenactment pressures. They may have difficulty keeping an objective appraisal of what is taking place, especially as they are learning the rules of the craft. The supervisor helps the trainee correct course and learn about the power and value of these pressures. In this chapter, I share the guidelines I have used as a supervisor in a psychiatry residency program.

Discovering Psychotherapy Patients

I was once told by an instructor, when I was inquiring about how to obtain psychoanalytic cases, "Psychoanalysis patients are not ready-made; they need to be discovered." He was, I believe, underlining something that also applies to therapy cases more generally. We should approach all patients with an openness to the immense scope of their subjectivity. Even when I was working in an outpatient setting that was ostensibly for medication management, I would educate *all* patients I saw about the benefits of psychotherapy. I would tell them that medications can undoubtedly be an important aid to help alleviate symptoms. However, to do justice to the complexity of what they were going through and to individualize the approach, regular meetings with a therapist could be very helpful. Of course, autonomy is always to be respected, and no one is ever to be forced to do therapy if it is not of interest. It is, after all, a process requiring an emotional, financial, and time commitment that may not always be feasible. Even if someone *does* wish to do therapy, the patient may not want to "dig into the past"; rather, the individual may want to discuss symptoms objectively and learn practical ways to address them. This also needs to be respected, because there is no "one size fits all" when it comes to therapy; we need to meet patients where they are. Even if the patient is interested in dynamic work, it does not mean that we throw out the need for supportive interventions and psychoeducation, particularly at the beginning of treatment.

If psychodynamic therapy is the agreed-upon modality, the commitment to weekly sessions (at the least) should, in my opinion, be stressed. Anything less frequent may turn the treatment into a series of "catch-up sessions." Therapy every 2 weeks, for instance, amounts to 100 minutes a month (for 50-minute sessions), which is under 2 hours. Although psychoanalysis typically warrants a frequency of three to five weekly sessions, a psychodynamic process can certainly be fostered by meeting once or twice a week. Maintaining a regular meeting time each week is highly encouraged because this allows patients to feel that that specific hour during the week is truly "theirs" (this will be elaborated upon in Chapters 3 and 11).

It is not uncommon for patients to work for a period of time in weekly therapy and, when they feel they are in a more "stable" place, to request a decrease in frequency to every other week or monthly. Therapists may agree to this rather readily, for some reason. My reaction is quite the opposite: if someone is feeling more stable, perhaps this indicates that deeper work can be more safely engaged in, allowing us to consider *increasing* the frequency to capitalize on the gains garnered thus far. These are all matters the supervisor can discuss with the trainee during the initial portions of the academic year, when a caseload is inherited (from a graduating trainee) and initial sessions are being held.

Importantly, I think that there is often a "previous provider bias" when taking someone else's caseload. A patient might be signed out as, for instance, "Patient X, 30 years old, diagnosis of borderline personality disorder. Don't even try insight-oriented therapy; stick with supportive therapy and meds." It is remarkable how common such shorthand sign-outs actually are. This is a very reductionistic encapsulation, to say the least, which effectively dismisses the potential for actual depth work to be done. It is a despairing situation for patients when their doctor has given up on them. I always encourage residents to take a fresh look at patients, create their *own* diagnostic impressions, and wonder about how a patient's symptom spectrum and forms of relating, no matter *how* seemingly disturbed, make sense to the patient on some level of the psyche. It is our job to empathize with our patients' distress and understand why some maladaptive forms of relating may be *necessary*.

Current symptoms might stem from very early experiences, and we seek to explore with our patients how developmental factors may be contributing to issues in adulthood. Needless to say, this takes time, with patience from both parties being essential, especially because we need to be open and flexible to symptom *worsening* and feelings of stagnation in sessions.

Structuring the Supervisory Hour

For my supervisory hour, I request residents to bring in process notes on patients. It was a very useful experience for me during residency and psychoanalytic training to sit after a session and re-create the dynamics by way of a transcript. We are often swept up by the intensity of sessions and may have difficulty keeping our own thinking going during the hour. After it is over, it can be helpful to give ourselves space for quiet contemplation and for processing what just took place. In revisiting sessions and typing them out, we provide supervision to ourselves, in some ways, and can bring in our own impressions to our supervisors. I found that supervisors liked having a transcript printed out for them, and we would review the material line by line, paying close attention to the nuances of session dynamics. This allowed me to investigate how I communicated with my patients, how I guided them in productive ways or led them astray, and how my own interventions in sessions might have been subtle (or overt) forms of reenactment.

Guidance for process notes is straightforward—the transcription is verbatim (as much as possible), and residents can indicate moments of silence in sessions, a patient's shift in body language or facial expression, and *the resident's own* associations or emotional responses in particular moments (if they feel comfortable sharing them). For instance:

> T: I wonder how you're feeling.
> P: I'm not feeling anything.
> (Silence for 60 seconds; patient looked uncomfortable.)
> (I felt awkward, I broke the silence, not sure why but patient was staring intensely at me while I was quiet.)
> T: Nothing at all?

Using supervision in this way allows for an in-depth appreciation of session dynamics. It is very different from coming to a supervisory hour without a transcript and giving more general comments: "The patient came in late, got mad at me at one point....I think he talked about his mom. We then discussed meds, I think. He used an interesting word at one point, but it's gone now." It makes it difficult for both trainee and supervisor to navigate the hour without a map. The transcript can be grounding in this regard.

As discussed later in this book (see Chapters 3, 4, and 5), there is much to be gleaned from how sessions begin and end—how patients reintroduce themselves to us and how we cut off contact with them, respectively. I often make a point of discussing beginnings of sessions in supervision. Of note, it is crucial that transcripts be presented in all their crudeness (i.e., what is said should not be "cleaned up" to sound more sophisticated, insightful, or seamless). Therapy is difficult, it is messy, and patients are trying to describe something that can never be perfectly expressed through any combination of words. It is not helpful if the "um"s, "huh"s, "hmm"s, "like"s, and "I mean"s of the patient (or therapist, for that matter) are eliminated to "improve clarity" or (shudder) to impress the supervisor with how amazing the session was. This is anathema to the work and a lost opportunity to understand how such forms of communicating may be *necessary* in a given moment. As will be discussed, sometimes words are used to *undo* any chance of understanding taking place. By cleaning things up, we are attributing our own projected meaning onto the patient's communications, as opposed to looking at the "imperfections" in speech and the quizzical gaps as something of greater value than flawless elocution. In modifying the transcript as such, we might be participating in a form of reenactment because patients may have never found someone who was actually curious about what *they* had in mind but rather might have interacted with impatient individuals who gave their own take on matters and moved on. Such patients may have learned that their own minds are unwelcome and must give way to how others feel a situation should be thought about and interpreted. Thus, a gap in the flow of speech may represent a hope for this gap to be listened to for what it might *become* if treated with interest, as opposed to being seen as an inconvenience to be stopped up with meaningless filler. I do *not* recommend documenting or bringing to supervision every single word said in a session (as I emphasize below). However, the sections that *are* brought in should be as faithful as possible to what took place.

Taking Notes in Sessions

In terms of taking notes *during* sessions, advice varies widely. Nowadays, transcription apps have become popular (though they are far from error-free and can be unwieldy because an unedited transcript can run 15–20 pages, often with many typos and run-in phrases that mix the words of the therapist and patient). Other supervisees opt to take notes during sessions and then type up the content later. If one chooses the latter, it is *not* advisable to try to write down every word a patient says, for at least two reasons: 1) it is not possible to do so, and 2) it will detract from one's ability to engage more openly with patients if there is the need to concurrently pay attention to what is being written down. The therapist may choose to write "key" words or passages, serving as grounding markers to guide session reconstruction later. Of course, if one writes *anything* during a session, patients will (understandably) have feelings about things being written down about them. They may, for instance, develop a "pen transference," wherein they will be cognizant of what content the therapist deems "worthwhile" (vs. material that is not worth the bother). There may also be an expectation for us to be the repositories of past sessions. At times when I took notes, some patients would begin sessions with "Tell me where we left off." (Of course, this can be explored without a concrete answer being given.)

We do need to be transparent about where session material is being stored and whether what is being said in a session is going to be shared in supervision, with colleagues, or in notes in the medical record. Although we want to be open to patients' fantasies about what we do with said material, there does need to be concrete reassurance to patients that their confidentiality will not be violated, that material shared in supervision will be done so in a private setting for educational purposes, and that notes from sessions will be stored securely so that no one else will have access to them. Regarding medical records, it is not advisable to put long stretches of content into therapy notes but rather to do "abbreviated notes" for the record and to keep one's own "session notes" and transcripts for personal use and supervision. If a trainee chooses to audio record the session (facilitating transcription and playback of passages to the supervisor), explicit permission needs to be obtained from patients to do so; my recommendation is for the file to be erased after the subsequent supervisory hour has taken place.

Selecting a Case for Supervision

> *I have been thinking[…]that the social moulds civilization fits us into have no more relation to our actual shapes than the conventional shapes of the constellations have to the real star-patterns.*
>
> Thomas Hardy (1895/2016, p. 168)

In terms of selecting a patient for discussion, it makes intuitive sense for a trainee to present someone with a level of functioning permitting "insight-oriented" work, though what this means is not easily definable. Patients should 1) be able to commit to regular therapy, 2) have an interest in learning about themselves, 3) have the capacity to sit with difficult emotions without engaging in overtly destructive behaviors (which would limit our ability to maintain a therapeutic stance without resorting to more concrete interventions to prevent harm), 4) not have an impairment in reality testing that precludes abstract or symbolic thinking (if a patient is functioning on a psychotic level, dynamic therapy is usually not recommended, particularly for trainee therapists), 5) not be actively using licit or illicit substances to the point of impairing cognition, and 6) not be engaging in activities that warrant mandatory reporting to the authorities. We do not make blanket assumptions about a patient's suitability for treatment based on academic or vocational functioning, previous failure of psychotherapeutic trials, criminal history, unemployment, historical diagnoses (it is a sad reality in psychiatry that many times, a charted diagnosis is completely unreliable), socioeconomic status, or even a matter such as lacking stable housing.[1] Trainees should be encouraged to be open to the possibility of doing psychotherapy with *anyone* who comes for help as long as it is clinically appropriate and of interest to the patient. I have been astounded by the wonderful work some residents have done by engaging patients in productive psychodynamic therapy when previous providers had deemed the patients "inappropriate" for such a modality.

There may be some trial and error in finding a suitable case for supervision because some patients drop out of treatment or decide not to commit to a frequency allowing for sufficient continuity. Supervision can also be used for *figuring out* which patients might be a good choice for discussion, especially if the trainee is struggling with the selection. Once a decision is made and the work of supervision begins, it is a very rewarding process.

That said, I frequently wonder about the patients who are *not* discussed. It is a very common observation on the residents' parts that they feel they provide therapy of uneven quality to their patients. Namely, the ones being discussed in supervision have a much richer surround to them in terms of both attention and reflection. Several factors contribute to this. For these patients, residents will 1) spend a considerable amount of time on process notes, 2) think more deeply about their own interventions and countertransference, 3) anxiously (or supportively) hold the supervisor's voice in mind during sessions (feeling that pressure to "bring up that thing we discussed in supervision" to report back on how it went), 4) read articles and chapters pertaining more immediately to the patient in question, and 5) perhaps feel more invested in continuing work with the patient into another year of residency or training (if possible) or increasing the number of weekly sessions. In other words, it is almost like choosing a favorite child or having a "treatment group" and a "control group," one receiving more of an intensive psychodynamic intervention, while the other patients receive more supportive or hybrid forms of therapy. It has been sobering to inquire with residents about the patients

---

[1] For a compelling analysis of doing psychodynamic work with underserved and marginalized populations, readers are referred to the work by Berzoff (2012).

who have been kept *out* of the supervisory hour. Startlingly, some had uncanny childhood histories of never having experienced a place of their own, feeling lost in the household and deindividualized, and being brought up by parents who felt that giving them a roof and nourishment was enough (as we provide them with an office setting and an exchange of words for 50 minutes). Some of these patients reported feeling there was something more to them that was never cultivated, something that could have brought about a greater richness to life. In *not* choosing certain patients, we may unwittingly be reliving with them a powerful dynamic that speaks to a familiar form of treatment from early life. As Jerry Seinfeld observed, "Sometimes the road less traveled is less traveled for a reason." This is not to suggest that every single patient needs to have an individual supervisor (which is itself a topic worthy of discussion); rather it reflects a reality inherent to the structuring of the outpatient experience in many training programs. It would, naturally, be untenable and burnout-inducing for a trainee to expend such energy on each patient. In any event, seeing *all* patients as potential psychodynamic cases is a valid approach. This keeps us from foreclosing the possibility of doing meaningful, long-term work with someone who could very well benefit from it if given the chance.

I have found it an incredibly heartening and rewarding experience to have a resident struggling to make sense of a patient tell me, "This is not someone who one would usually think of as psychodynamic, but there seems to be so much there, so much to talk about, and I'd really like to take that approach to see where we go." And we do; we struggle together. The outcomes have been at times quite revelatory because the residents open themselves up to these individuals' life experiences in ways that have never been allowed before; they create space for wonder, as opposed to reinforcing the well-trodden worldly response of shutting things down with exasperated, impatient shortness. *Everyone* has a subjectivity worth knowing, and empathy will never go out of style. Every patient is worth the fight.

The Supervisor's Approach

What supervisors impart to trainees will be informed by their experience, theoretical inclinations, and technical approach. Trainees may feel the pressure to "conform" to certain ways of thinking about and interacting with patients. This is counter to the fostering of an individuality in trainees, to allowing their own style of relating to patients to emerge. As supervisors, we are not trying to create replicas of ourselves. I make sure to tell residents that *they* are the ones in the room with the patients and that they need to feel comfortable incorporating particular topics into the fabric of the sessions. And when they do so, they should feel empowered to do so using their *own* words, conveying ideas we discuss in supervision in the ways they feel work best for individual patients. There is the phenomenon of "Monday morning quarterbacking" that can take place in supervision, wherein it seems as though the supervisor has a Jedi-like insight into the issues at hand, always with the perfect response that ties up everything nicely. This is simply not the case. Being in the room is completely different because it carries with it the intensity of the patients' emotional worlds, impacting how the therapist thinks and behaves. It is the supervisory hour that can allow for a joint processing of such dynamics; it gives some breathing room in which one can calmly think alongside an experienced other and reflect on what happened during the session. Trainees often have the feeling of missed opportunities or of having said something silly that moved them away from important content. It is crucial for trainees not to hold themselves up to impossible standards. Working with patients on this level is very difficult. As we grapple with material that can be very unsettling, words may fail us; we might choose the wrong ones; empathic breaks can occur; we may remain too much on the surface; we might extend beyond 50 minutes and violate the frame. In supervision, we gently and thoughtfully pay attention to what took place and try to understand it in light of transference-countertransference dynamics. It is all grist for exploration.

Insights from the supervisory hour will be taken with the trainee into the next session, and the lens will thus be slightly different, which can lead to small shifts. For instance, perhaps the therapist allows for some instances of silence, whereas before, such quiet moments would be anxiety-provoking and broken with a "clarifying" question or statement. Perhaps the trainee will find a way to speak to some transference-related topic in a session, providing a chance to observe how the patient negotiates such an intervention. This is the continued work of supervision, which gives trainees the experience of gaining an in-depth understanding of a particular patient, as well as how *their own* minds evolve over the course of the year. Trainees will experience themselves as real and transference-distorted objects in patients' lives, feeling pressured to relive internalized templates and finding ways to bring such dynamics to their patients' awareness, all in an effort to transform something viscerally felt into something that can be articulated and understood in new ways.

Engaging With Readings

As a form of supplementing the supervisory experience, I have made a habit of giving residents reading assignments each week. Typically, we spend 10 minutes discussing the reading followed by 40–45 minutes discussing the patient and going over process notes. Some of the readings, particularly at the beginning, may seem esoteric or difficult to apply clinically. (After all, what is being learned is a new way of thinking about patients, many of the principles of which are not intuitive.) What I suggest to residents is to let the material "wash over" them and see what resonates. I suggest they extract *one clinically relevant idea* from each reading. In no way is it expected that residents will be able to make perfect sense of a psychodynamic or psychoanalytic paper, because even very experienced clinicians and scholars could pore over works and derive a number of different conclusions from them.

My experience has been that if residents maintain the discipline of reading assigned papers, the knowledge base acquired by the end of the academic year is tremendous. What is read will become increasingly salient to their clinical work. The incorporation of reading material also allows for the development of critical thinking and an evolution of one's individual therapeutic stance, as opposed to shaping one's mind in accordance with the supervisor's point of view. I opt for works that are readable and digestible in 1 week, usually around 10–20 pages. With each reading, it is important for there to be a discussion about how these concepts are applicable to real-world therapy. Some lines from readings need to be said aloud, pondered over, tossed aside, read again, or yelled at. Most critically, these ideas need to be *thought about together*.

For interested readers, I have published elsewhere an annotated bibliography with a list of 32 sequential readings that can be incorporated over the academic year into the supervisory hour (Miller et al. 2019). However, there is no unassailable list. Rather, I believe it is the discipline of actively engaging the psychoanalytic literature along with the trainee that is the most helpful practice. I have also found that for individual residents, the lists of papers covered over the course of the year vary because I do not draw from a static selection but rather try to titrate what is assigned in accordance with relevant clinical concepts that pertain to the case we have been discussing. This has been a welcome approach by residents and has helped deepen their work with patients. Many educators have their own set of foundational readings; for this process to work, supervisors will want to assign works they are familiar with (or willing to discover alongside the trainee).

Personal Therapy

As a final note, I will briefly discuss the matter of trainees being in personal treatment. Despite popular belief, the notion of the therapist as a blank slate has increasingly fallen out of favor. Patients will inevitably have a strong effect on us. While we are real humans in the room, we need to avoid being unduly influenced by our own issues; patients come to us for help, and we should be attentive to how our own unresolved conflicts might interfere

with our being present therapeutically. This is why personal therapy is a
wonderful endeavor to pursue, both in training and beyond. For one, it allows us to understand what it is like to be in the patient's place and just how
difficult it is to be the one talking. Perhaps more important, it affords us a
space to concurrently discuss our own conflicts with a third party; providing
psychotherapy can be very challenging because we share the burden of our
patients' emotional turmoil. We leave work, but we take our minds with us,
and much of what happened in the room may stick with us. Being in personal therapy allows for a sharing of *our* struggles as well and is a form of
self-care.

It is *not* recommended to use a supervisor for discussing personal issues.
Supervisors are not meant to be therapists for trainees; rather, they are intended to be experienced advisors who help illustrate conflictual areas in patients' lives and how these may be revealing themselves in sessions. As I
mentioned in the introduction to this book, there are two object worlds interacting with each other during any clinical encounter. The goal in supervision is to understand what aspects of the *patient's* internal object world
may be presenting in the fabric of sessions. This is not the full picture—nor
could it be, lest we place an unfair burden on our patients, as though what is
taking place is *entirely* a reliving of their internal worlds, disavowing the role
our own subjectivity might have played in facilitating or inhibiting certain
dynamics. Through personal treatment, therapists can process how their *own*
internal object worlds may be influencing sessions with particular patients.
This two-pronged approach to understanding the intersection of two distinct object worlds can greatly enhance the therapeutic work we do.

KEY POINTS

- Engaging in psychotherapy supervision is a critical component in
  one's development as a therapist.

- Within the object relations model, our internal world interacts
  with that of the patient. Given the potential for identifying with our
  patients' projections (leading to reenactments), an outside observer with whom one can process session content is key to identifying dynamics that are being relived in sessions.

- The addition of psychoanalytic literature to the supervisory hour
  can help expose a trainee to new ideas and consolidate their clinical relevance, particularly with regard to the patient(s) being discussed.

References

Berzoff J: Falling Through the Cracks: Psychodynamic Practice With Vulnerable and Oppressed Populations. New York, Columbia University Press, 2012

Hardy T: Jude the Obscure (1895). Norton Critical Edition. New York, WW Norton, 2016

Hesse H: The Glass Bead Game (1943). New York, Picador, 2012

Miller CWT, Hodzic V, Ross DR, Ehrenreich MJ: Annotated bibliography for supervising psychiatry residents in psychodynamic psychotherapy. Acad Psychiatry 43(4):417–424, 2019 30997655

Establishing and Maintaining a Therapeutic Frame

[I]t is the very steadiness of the framework which permits the "freedom" of free association to take place in a meaningful rather than an anarchic way.

Allannah Furlong (1992, p. 705)

ONE OF THE MOST important aspects of psychodynamic therapy is establishing and maintaining a therapeutic frame. It gives us mental scaffolding, keeping us grounded in the midst of uncertainty. When I speak of the frame, I am referring to the very practical aspects of the treatment—where we meet, for how long, on what day(s), where I will sit and where the patient can sit, whether I will be discussing session material with a supervisor, what happens to my notes (or audio recordings, if applicable), whether there is a stop date for our work (a common reality in training programs), and many others. We need to be transparent about these matters because both the therapist and patient come to rely on them as nonnegotiables that ground the treatment in something safe and sturdy.

In this chapter, I will expand on several dimensions relating to the therapeutic frame. I start by commenting on a conspicuous *absence* from my discussion—the matter of the fee. Although it is a very important aspect of the frame, this book is mostly geared toward conducting therapy in educational or training settings, where billing patients and handling money are inconsistently negotiated elements of care (they may even be absent in some programs). This may be due to fees being waived given the learner status of trainees or because the providers are in clinics where billing is handled through administrative staff (in some instances, insurance may cover the cost entirely, with *no* co-pay for patients). In other words, the reality can be very different from that of therapists working in private practice settings. I refer interested readers to some of the extant literature on the importance of the fee (Allen 1971; Furlong 1992; Myers 2008; Pauley 2019).

The Therapeutic Frame

The frame is sacred. It is the foundation upon which we establish the parameters of our availability to patients. It is the inescapable reminder of our separateness and of our limitations. We have a start time and stop time to which we adhere. Patients are encouraged to speak about anything they like, but the relationship is restricted to verbal forms of expression, and its intimacy never goes beyond what is strictly professional. When patients are ensured a setting in which they can feel secure of the boundaries in place, they are freed up to speak about the most disturbing, titillating, and provocative content that goes through their minds, knowing that the ones listening will not compromise this process by impinging their own needs and desires onto their patients.

Time

When beginning treatment, I always recommend establishing a clear time allotment for the duration of sessions and sticking with it. It should be clear to patients whether sessions will be 45, 50, 55, or 60 minutes and that the therapist will be stopping at the mark (or sometime within those last 60 seconds). Of note, in this chapter, I have chosen 50 minutes as a standard duration for sessions because this is what I follow.

As we invite our patients to immerse themselves in the exploration process, we do so in a warm and flexible manner, knowing that it will end at a predictable time. While they are with us, the time is theirs; we will listen to their words attentively and take what they are saying seriously. We open space for further exploration as much as possible. However, no therapist can be endlessly available. We help patients access and sit with challenging thoughts and emotions, as sessions often veer in unexpected directions, but there must always be a reality component to keep both parties grounded. Reality is always a force to be negotiated in our lives, as much as we may wish to depart from its constraints. This applies to healing even in the most introspective of settings. On some spiritual retreats, the periods dedicated to meditation are often ended at one point by the softness of a chime or by a gong. Time is up. Although the meditation practice is over, the places people accessed in their minds will be carried forward until the next meditative experience, wherein perhaps even greater depths will be reached. Similarly, what is taken from one psychotherapy session will be elaborated on in the patient's mind throughout the week, in moments of quiet, in interactions with others, in dreams, and in further insights and associations stemming from what happened during the past session. When the next session arrives, the work continues. It never really stopped because the unconscious is always active. This perspective may help limit the pressure a therapist feels to address everything on the patient's mind in the span of one session (or even over the course of an entire treatment, no matter how intensive and prolonged).

Sometimes there is reluctance to end on time if the patient is bringing up "good material." This is where the "process versus content" question becomes important (discussed in Chapter 5, "Finding the Focus: Content Versus Process"). If a patient is bringing up something that seems very pressing right at the end of the session, we may imagine there is a communicative function to it beyond what the content reveals. The patient may wish to draw us in, extend the session, and have it become something *other* than a provider-patient relationship with clear rules. Attempts to keep going past the end mark may be a protest against the frame and a desire to remain in the therapist's mind after the session ends. The therapist may experience guilt for "being inflexible" or "dropping the patient when I was needed the most." In some instances, we can understand these pressures as a patient needing to eliminate a sense of separateness when reality demands it. The therapist, in this moment, might be experienced as cold and depriving. Rather than capitulating, it is important to gently let the patient know that what is being said is of great import and that it can be discussed during the next session, perhaps even saying that to do justice to what is being said, more time is *necessary*, and rushing through it is cheating it of its importance.

Notably, tension and irritability can arise in the therapist when the minute strikes for the session to end and it feels there is no way to stop the patient's associations. Empathy struggles with the clock in such moments, and it suddenly becomes a burden to continue having this individual in the room; the patient is "impinging" on the therapist's right to alone time, to write a note, to attend to other patients, and to deal with many other obligations (which become all the more pressing as the patient continues to talk). I refer to this as "51st-minute empathy," wherein our patience and benign stance seem to drain away in direct proportion to the passing of the seconds once 50 minutes hits. The type of object the patient *becomes* to us in those moments beyond the "time is up" strike of the clock can help us understand, in very visceral ways, how particular object relationship templates may be reenacted. Perhaps the patient experienced having caregivers who only provided attention for a set time before turning to "more important matters," leaving the child with a vivid feeling of being an inconvenience to the caregivers, who would only show empathy or love for a limited time, on their own terms. In pushing the bounds of the frame, we may be pressured by our patients to relive this role of an impatient caregiver who wants to shoo away the needy child. When a therapist ends a session, it can feel like a hateful and aggressive act because it introduces total physical separation until the next meeting. The British pediatrician and psychoanalyst Donald Winnicott stated, "Hate is expressed by the existence of the end of the 'hour'" (Winnicott 1949, p. 71). The reality of needing to end sessions on time and what this means for the patient and therapist are grist for exploration. Although frustrating, it is also necessary, and knowing there are clear guardrails in place can help patients relax into the short-lived "timelessness" of sessions without the anxiety of being pulled into the unpredictability of the exploration and losing the reassurance that "ordinary reality" brings.

There are advantages to a certain "roughness" at the ends of sessions, as opposed to tying up things neatly. Trainees sometimes feel pressured to provide a summary or recap of "take-home points" from the session, almost turning the encounter into a single-standing event that could exist on its own, apart from the other single sessions. Instead, it is useful to foster an evolving narrative that is *not* self-contained but rather an opening up of space to further the work beyond the limits of the 50 minutes. Ending a session in a state of unfinished business—of suspension—invites more of a "what's next" feel, allowing the patient to feel a bit unsettled when leaving the room, thinking about what was said (and left unsaid) during the encounter. Importantly, further associations and the manifold goings-on of the unconscious over the course of the following days will influence what is overtly on the patient's mind at the start of the next meeting. We encourage this mind to give itself freedom of expression, a slow and delicate process that often undoes the "certainties" previously held to, creating space for grayness.

At times, communication within sessions is less important than what happens in the periods before and after meeting. Patients may feel overwhelmed and pressured when coming into the office, feeling it is all on them to produce content. Sometimes there is a lot to say, and they clam up when in front of us, unable to convey their internal state through words. On our end, the things we say to patients may fall flat in a session, or patients may simply not be in a place to process them while in our presence. It is a very common phenomenon to say something that, to us, makes *perfect* sense yet seems like a foreign language to the patient. When this happens, we might feel deflated, incompetent, or even angry; however, in certain instances, patients simply need time to make sense of what we have said, on *their* terms, sometimes on their own, away from us. It is not uncommon for a patient to come back the following week, or indeed months later, saying, "You know, I've thought about what you said some time ago, and it really makes sense. I wasn't ready to hear it when you said it, but it stuck with me, and I was able to think about it more."

Ultimately, there is a kindness behind maintaining a clear and reliable frame. We recognize that we as therapists have limitations and respect what sessions can realistically provide to patients within 50-minute spans. We are not omniscient creatures who can deliver immediate and all-encompassing insights. We meet patients with the minds we *do* have, knowing we are setting something in motion without a clear destination in mind, with openness and patience to brave the journey together.

Just as we need to be mindful of ending sessions on time, we also need to be prepared to *start* on time. We want patients to feel that the time set aside each week is reliably and predictably theirs. This is one of the arguments for trying to establish a set time each week for a particular patient, as opposed to changing times from one week to the next. Although patients may show up late for appointments, which will, of course, be something important to think about and discuss, we need to hold ourselves accountable for our own punctuality. It is much more feasible to attempt to discuss what led a patient to show up late for a given session than to process what is causing *us* to fail to be ready to work with this individual at the agreed-upon time. A therapist who is unable to maintain a frame may be experienced as an unreliable object. Patients need to have a sense of our sturdiness in order to allow themselves to be vulnerable in our presence.

Part of this sturdiness is holding in mind how patients treat the start time of sessions. Some patients are reliably on time, and some are reliably late. Either way, it is important to understand for each patient what the meaning is of how the allotted 50 minutes are negotiated. Perhaps the therapist is experienced as having all the control and "dictating" every aspect of a unilateral relationship, one in which the patient shoulders all the physical, emotional, and financial burden. Showing up consistently late *takes back* some control and keeps the therapist in the role of the one waiting for and thinking about the patient. In effect, a therapist waiting for a late patient is paralyzed from really doing anything else; therapy cannot take place, and other endeavors would only be taken up in tense ways, perhaps even with a feeling of transgression on the part of the therapist, who may feel as though checking an email or picking up a newspaper would be akin to putting a hand in the cookie jar, risking being caught by the patient rushing through the door and catching the sneaky therapist in the act. During these minutes of lateness, there is something of an inversion of the power differential; it is one of the few concrete elements that patients control regarding the frame. If a patient shows up late and the therapist still ends the session at the 50-minute mark (which I believe needs to be enforced), the total time will be shortened, and we will need to explore with patients why it is that they do not (or *cannot*) allow themselves to have their full 50 minutes.

It is also useful to explore with patients what type of therapist-object they expect to encounter in the office when they walk in past the set start time. Just as we are different people at minute 51, who we become when we are kept waiting may be, in the mind of the patient (and perhaps in reality), *very* different from who we were some minutes earlier, prior to lateness being a factor. In instances when patients have an expectation of us turning into angry and impatient figures, showing up late can be a way of testing the waters and nudging us toward *becoming* such figures because they might imagine we become testier as the seconds go by. A patient, after showing up late, may uncharacteristically ask, "How are you?" In my mind, I'm translating this question as "Are you going to kill me?" Whether the question of how I am relates or not to lateness on a conscious level (and indeed, we can be accused of "reading too much into" what patients say), what is undeniable is that this question is being asked *in the context* of lateness. Thus, this aspect needs to be taken into account when we think about the meaning of the question.

There are many times when patients may feel that we only tolerate them because they play according to our rules, do not rock the boat too much, and do not overtly express hostile feelings toward us. During such smooth forms of relating, one wonders where the aggressive impulses lie and why they cannot find their way into the sessions. Dropping us for a few minutes can be a less direct (though quite overt) manifestation of such urges. The aggressiveness might be projected into *us*, generating the expectation that we will react angrily to them. If we identify with this projection, we may indeed find ourselves *becoming* annoyed with the patient, feeling the latter is being passive-aggressive and wasting our time. Sometimes in an attempt to neutralize any feeling of hostility in ourselves (as opposed to understanding the type of object relationship being lived in the here and now), we push the projection away and reassure both ourselves and the patient there is no aggressiveness to be found. Thus, we might respond "Good" to the question of how we are doing, or we may allow ourselves to be convinced by patients' explanations of how, before *every* session, there is some major traffic inconvenience, roadwork, emergency phone call, or other interfering life event that precludes arriving to appointments on time. If we collude that there is no psychological meaning to the patient's lateness, we risk missing something important that is being relived in the transference-countertransference, something demanding to be seen (through its repetition each session) yet covered over by superficial explanations. Perhaps this is the only way that a particular dynamic or conflict *can* make itself known, and all it requires of us is to be attentive to the frame and think together with our patients about why it is being impinged upon.

One of my very first therapy patients had the habit of always being 10 minutes late for sessions. Despite encouragement from my supervisor, I was very hesitant to bring it up with her, for fear she would become upset and leave. This went on for about 6 months. During one session, I brought it up, stating, "You know, I've noticed I'm the only one here for the first 10 minutes of our sessions." She looked at me with wide eyes, startled. She began tearing up and said, "Why are you only saying this *now*? I've been coming here for months, and you've never brought it up. I ended up thinking, 'Oh, he must like it that I never show up on time. He can't deal with me for a whole 50 minutes. I'll just keep doing it….' And you never said anything, so I figured my theory was right. I know I'm a handful." This flooded me with guilt over not having mentioned it before, because I was implicitly affirming to her by not discussing her lateness that I did not care to have her any longer than I absolutely needed to and that her recurring lateness was a welcome relief from the misery of hearing about her internal world. This exemplifies how exploring how patients negotiate the start time gives us a glimpse into internalized relationship templates; ignoring a patient's handling of the frame may be unwittingly casting us into the role of a neglectful caregiver, which can have very destructive effects. We must remember that there is no such thing as a session that starts late. *Every* session starts on time; sometimes the therapist just happens to be the only one in the room.

Discussing lateness is not easy, and when tardiness is a recurring factor, it can feel like we are being annoying by insisting on talking about what it means. We end up identifying as the ones who assign value and importance to having a full session, while patients might be content to dismiss its significance and keep the meaning of lateness in the realm of concrete busyness and traffic matters. They might even feel irritated with us if we "keep bringing up lateness," as though we are making a big deal of something trivial, cutting into the time to discuss more important topics. We may feel guilty and collude with what the patient is saying. It ends up feeling as though we are delaying the start of the "real session" even more by harping on those lost minutes. It can be useful to think of it as follows: it is not the therapist who keeps bringing up lateness; rather, it is the patient who does, by continuing to show up late. And, crucially, it is *being* brought up because it *needs* to be spoken to, as uncomfortable as this might be for both individuals in the room.

A somewhat similar philosophy can apply to patients who seem to be on time almost to the point of obsessiveness. Some arrive 30 or 60 minutes early, sitting in the waiting room, sometimes in clear sight of the therapist, who may be transiting in and out. (This might indicate they *want* to be seen and kept in the mind of their therapist even before the session begins. They could just as easily have stayed in the car or in the building lobby.) As suggested, arriving late can be a way of "poking the beast" by angering the therapist. For other patients, however, it can be terribly anxiety-provoking to imagine coming to a session even 1 minute late, lest they encounter an intolerant and hateful object that allows for *no* deviation from the frame, no matter the circumstances. If a patient has come to hundreds of sessions and has *never* been tardy, I would wonder what the significance of this is in the patient's mind and what it would mean to arrive late. When I broached this topic with a very punctual patient, he said, "It's hard for me to even think of. When I try to imagine it, I'm consumed with some blinding sound [sic] in my head....I think my brain would fall apart."

The Clock

While therapists need to have access to a clock to be sure sessions start and stop on time, it is a matter of debate whether patients should be able to see the clock during encounters. There are pluses and minuses to patients knowing how much time is left. My position is that it is preferable for patients not to have a clock visible during sessions, and I elaborate on my reasoning in this section.

One disadvantage to being able to see a clock is that sometimes patients censor themselves if they feel there is not enough time to address a particular issue. Some of the most important material can emerge when they are immersed in free association, not burdened by minute counting; even if they bring up something very traumatic with 1 minute to spare, perhaps that is all that can be accessed during that session, though much remains unsaid. However, it might not have been spoken of *at all* if they thought time was too limited. Similarly, I advise against making statements such as "We only have 5 minutes left, so maybe we shouldn't start anything too deep right now" or "Let's recap our session during these few minutes." Just as we can learn from how patients begin sessions, much is to be learned from how they react to our ending sessions, without too much preemptive padding. I have also come to believe that many patients, on some level, can sense when time is coming to a close. In some instances, this can result in a "shutting down" or turning to banal matters or posing to the therapist, "I don't think we have much time left. Maybe we should stop early." One may see this as an attempt to summon up the defenses needed to go back out into the world, as opposed to remaining in a state of emotional vulnerability and then suddenly having the session terminated by a clock-watching therapist. It brings back some level of control to the patient's side. Our clock or watch may also become a persecutory element in the room because it is a never-ending reminder of a reality that will always carry us away from our patients. A female patient, when I said that time was up, sat up and looked at her watch. She said, "You know, it's only 3:49. [It was 3:50 according to my clock.] We have 1 minute left. You stole a minute from me." She refused to look at my clock, which was in her sights when she sat up. Rather, she stared at me and brought up her wrist to show me her watch. At the beginning of the next session, before lying on the couch, she gave me a wry smile and asked, "Is your watch a good boy today? It was a bad, bad watch last time." I reflected back, "Maybe it's a 'good watch' when it's synched up with you. It becomes a bad watch when it doesn't work the way you want it to, keeping time according to its own schedule. Maybe it's the same with me—I'm good as long as I don't tell you our session is over, since you may feel otherwise, depending on how much you need our time together to go on." She laughed and said, "Let me see that clock of yours. Okay, we have the same time today."

As alluded to earlier, as sessions are nearing the end, patients might bring in very loaded material, deciding at that time to discuss a horrific dream, a past traumatic experience that has never been discussed before, or some important transference issue. There are many ways to interpret such situations. As mentioned, it might be an attempt to efface the frame, blurring the separateness between the therapist and patient. Such a dynamic is also present when patients take an inordinately long time to get up, very slowly collect their belongings, mention they need multiple medication refills, or pull out their planners to confirm future sessions (even if no confirmation is ostensibly needed because of the regularity of the encounters). We recognize that there is something very painful about leaving the room in the present state of mind, and remaining with us for as long as possible is a form of self-preservation, lest they feel something needed is being summarily torn away. We can notice these attempts at maintaining proximity both with the ends of sessions and with scheduled vacations. When I mentioned to one patient that I was going to be away for a week in the upcoming month, she looked at her calendar, and her face suddenly lit up—"You *are? That* week? So am *I*!! I'll be going on a hiking trip. We're on vacation together! I'll see you up on the mountain!" This fantasy undoes the need for separateness, uniting us beyond the limits of the session, in an ethereal space far above the common ground of reality.

As suggested earlier, another way to understand why patients might bring up very salient material toward the end of a session is that they are giving us a peek into important matters. Such topics can perhaps only be accessed in piecemeal and truncated ways, when there is not the risk of having too much time for exploration, which might feel *too* exposing. Bringing such topics up at the end is a way to "drop the crumb," which will remain in the minds of both individuals in the room. (Whether it will be brought up again in the next session or left up to the therapist to do so is always a hanging question.)

Abstinence and Neutrality

The term *abstinence* was used by Sigmund Freud as one of the parameters for conducting psychoanalysis (Freud 1919/1955). It was his position that a patient's active symptoms derive in part from warded-off instinctual impulses that are seeking satisfaction, which may take the form of a desire to gratify these wishes through the transference and the person of the therapist or analyst. Abstinence will facilitate exploration of the origins and deeper meanings behind these wishes, as opposed to being pulled into satisfying them through transference enactments.[1]

We can think of *neutrality* as maintaining an openness to what is happening in the patient's mind, as opposed to siding with a particular take on matters, which may be informed by an identification with projective pressures[2] or by a therapist's need in the moment to push one's own subjective viewpoint onto the patient. The term *anonymity* has also been used to refer to a therapist's lack of self-disclosure (Auchincloss and Samberg 2012), fostering ambiguity in the service of allowing patients to express their own reactions to and fantasies about the transference, as opposed to limiting them through too much "real-life" information.

These parameters are crucial to the integrity of the therapeutic space. While asserting the frame may be frustrating, it also reassures patients that things will not go too far, that an inappropriate permissiveness or intrusiveness on the therapist's part will not interfere with the potential for meaning-

---

[1] As stated by Greenson (1967), "The prolonged frustration will induce the patient to regress, so that his entire neurosis will be re-experienced in the transference, the transference neurosis. However, allowing symptom-substitute gratifications of any magnitude, in or outside of the analytic situation, will rob the patient of his neurotic suffering and his motivations to continue treatment" (pp. 275–276).

[2] In "The Ego and the Mechanisms of Defence," Anna Freud (1936) spoke of the analyst's need to remain in an "equidistant" position from a patient's ego, id, and superego.

ful work to be done. This is one reason why we should avoid bringing our own reality into sessions and, instead, maintain a focus on our patients' perspectives (including their thoughts on what we *might* be thinking or what they *imagine* to be true about our life outside the office). Sometimes there is a common historical fact between patient and therapist (e.g., trauma, divorced parents, or death of a sibling), and the temptation may arise for the latter to disclose this. This might appeal to the therapist as a way of strengthening the alliance—normalizing the patient's struggles with the reassurance that "I can relate." However, in doing so, we are cheating patients of the right for the therapy to be exclusively about *them*, and we risk overly aligning how patients "must be feeling" about their experiences with how we feel about ours (and vice versa). Although on the surface some events might have a degree of similarity, the impact may be completely different; we do not want to assume that patients do not need to elaborate any further on the effects of life events because it is taken for granted that we understand what they have been through. This can short-circuit important associations patients have to their own life histories, snared by the notion that common backgrounds imply common reactions and trajectories. Also, once it is brought into the room that the therapist has had "x" happen in the past, it might become the expectation that further information will be shared on request. Patients who learn of their therapists' life stories may, instead of thinking of their *own* reactions to their own unique life events, default to "How did *you* handle it when your sibling died?" It becomes a difficult situation to negotiate and hard for the therapist to say "Well, it's *your* hour, so why don't we focus on *you*?" when this was not the rule that was followed when the disclosure took place. A female patient whose brother had died when she was 9 years old had been previously seeing a female therapist who had a personal history of losing a sibling at a young age, which was promptly revealed by the therapist and led the patient to gravitate toward working with her for several months. However, as the work progressed, the patient discovered the space for processing her own loss was becoming increasingly diminished by the therapist's need to use the patient in a similar manner, discussing her own difficulties and turning the patient into someone suddenly impinged upon by a demanding object who had initially assumed the guise of being the one in the helping position. The therapy ended on this sour note.

Although we try to adhere to sound technique, sometimes we do self-disclose, even unwittingly. Such moments need not be viewed as irreparable breaches in the integrity of the work but rather are opportunities for exploration. I might say, "You know, I've been thinking about it. I noticed that I answered that question about my religion pretty directly and didn't really give us the chance to think about why it was coming up. I'm wondering if you have thoughts about how I handled that." I am not letting myself off the hook with regard to the reenactment but rather attempting to make therapeutic use of the moment to help us gain further insight.

The logic applied to self-disclosure can also be used with regard to giving advice. As our work with certain patients progresses, we often develop strong opinions about the ways they are "messing up their lives," believing they should make life choices according to what *we* think is best. We may have a blaring noise in our heads shouting, "Why don't you *just* [fill in the blank]???" (e.g., leave your spouse, quit your job, move, stop giving your kids money if they are misusing it, stop drinking so much to feel numb). It all seems so simple to us sometimes, and we have trouble figuring out why our patients do not just stop doing things that are seemingly so troubling and running counter to a healthier life. In some instances, we might be drawn into actually voicing these things. (It is far from uncommon for therapists to provide very concrete advice on things that they think their patients should be doing.) Giving advice bypasses learning what has led patients to make the choices they *have* made, instead of those seemingly simple, obvious, and revolutionary ones going through our minds. If the solution were that simple, it is unlikely patients would ever have made their way to therapy in the first place. After all, few (if any) of us have a firm grasp of what makes *us* function the way we do and what informs the choices we make. If we cannot figure out how to seamlessly navigate our own lives, can we really imagine we know what is best for someone we have seen for a rather limited amount of time and in a controlled setting? Patients will lead us to their knots, and it is not for us to try to undo them but rather to understand how they came to be, realize how they are indeed a *solution* in a way, and empathize with the need for them to exist. Untying them is hardly the goal. In many ways, the greater containment comes from patients' feeling that they have been heard and that we are not judging sensitive areas of their lives as something that needs to be concretely modified at all costs.

When I was a resident, a supervisor told me, "Get over your need to help your patient." Although it may seem cruel on some level, there is much wisdom in the notion of "getting over" the idea of quickly fixing matters. There is no quick fix. Taking this approach helps us relax in sessions, allowing better access to our own minds and improving the quality of the work. If we pollute the scene with pressures to find some resolution based on an incomplete understanding of a situation, we might be confirming some patients' deep-seated fears that there is no possibility of being fully listened to and understood by anyone. As a result, they may come to hate their own emotional state, as it has been shown to be something without a home in *any* mind. It is a privilege to be given access to a mind of endless complexity; we should not presume to know its machinations but rather surrender to its mystery. As Betty Joseph stated, "The analyst is fortunate in being given the opportunity to experience his impotence" (Joseph 1983, p. 296).

I wish to return to the idea of empathizing with the places in life patients find themselves in. Whatever unhealthy decisions patients might be making in terms of how they live their lives, these choices were made for reasons that, on *some* level in their minds, make perfect sense. To act differently would be to invite an anxiety too overwhelming to bear; bad choices are preferable to catastrophic ones. For instance, leaving an abusive spouse can certainly be seen as a healthier alternative to living with one and enduring the mistreatment. However, such a simplification ignores the reasons leading the person to stay. Individuals remain attached to people who treat them poorly for a variety of reasons. Children who suffer early abuse may identify with the motivations of their aggressors, feeling responsible for the abuse, and internalize this model of relating to others (at times in the active/abuser role) (Ferenczi 1949). Finding a way of reliving this dynamic in relationships can provide some sense of familiarity; after all, the alternative is not necessarily a healthy, benign relationship (which may never have been modeled and thus is thought of by the patient as an abstract construct that does not exist in reality) but rather a chaotic, groundless, and despairingly lonely world. If we adopt the position that patients should walk away from structures that are in place simply because we do not agree with them, we are in a way aligning ourselves with the abusers who valued their own subjectivity over that of the patient and wish to force the latter to adhere to our point of view. We may even become angry and frustrated when this does not happen, perhaps even wanting to snap at the patient and say, "If you're not going to listen to me, you clearly don't want help. Why are you even here?" In such instances, through projective identification, we have been drawn into the template of abuser-abused (in more subtle form, but still). Rather, it is more helpful to empathize with our patients about how difficult it must be to imagine themselves in a relationship *other* than one in which they are being abused and that there is something very powerful keeping them in it.

On our part, we hope to model a different form of object relationship with our patients, one in which *their* subjective experiences are not to be diminished by anyone else's. This allows patients to experience being treated differently, perhaps even taking in (introjecting) this function and treating themselves better as well. This would exemplify an updating of their internal object world through benign interactions with the therapist. In the process, we join in the struggle; we show patients we are willing to sit with them in the mire, understanding the paralysis and knowing there is not an easy way out. We show we can tolerate such paralysis, and, in doing so, we get a better idea of the place the patient lives in psychically. We need to relax into it and not just try to resolve it. As Gabbard (2009) stated, "Thinking about analysis as a remover of symptoms places an undue burden on the treatment. Some symptoms (e.g., certain forms of anxiety) are essential signals of inner turmoil. We can't do without them" (p. 585). I will now present two clinical vignettes to illustrate my reflections on the therapeutic frame.

Clinical Vignettes

Vignette 1

I was walking to my office to do paperwork one day (I had no appointments scheduled), and I encountered one of my therapy patients waiting for me, standing outside the locked door looking at her phone. While I was greeted with a smile and a familiar "hello," I was unsettled and questioning my own mind. I knew we did not have a session scheduled for that day, yet she was now expecting something from me that I was not prepared to give her. I openly questioned, "Do we have a session today?" (The very fact that I posed it in such a way is revelatory of my own wobbly commitment to maintaining the frame in that moment.) She realized that she was there on the wrong day, that our next session that week was really the next day, and she stated she would go back home (which was some distance away) and come back in the morning. I paused, thinking, "It's actually easier for me to see her now...." Based on this momentary reflection (or lack thereof), I told her I would see her right then. She hesitated for a moment, making sure I was actually sure I could, then came in. It is of note that this was on a Monday, after a weekend break, which perhaps led to her unconsciously attempting to close the gap between us. This would have been a worthwhile discussion point the next day, had I observed the integrity of the frame and explored how frustrating it must feel, as opposed to concretely shifting it through my impetuousness.

The session felt *very* off, as though we were living in a forbidden and alien space (which was indeed the case). She spoke very little, and I noticed myself saying trite, unhelpful things to her to try to free up her associations.

> P: I'm not sure I'm making any sense today....I had a dream last night, but I can't remember it, or my mind is telling me to keep it to myself.
> T: Maybe I can't be trusted in the same way today. It's harder to express yourself, since it may feel like we're not really supposed to be here.
> P: You were being nice....But maybe it would have been better for you to have turned me away. I don't like it here right now.

She had learned that I was not able to keep my own boundaries and mind intact when facing the pressures of her trying to find her way in. Once inside my mind, she was no longer in the presence of a reliable individual who could be trusted to contain and help her understand her inner world; rather, she was with someone of whom she should be suspicious, a therapist with a fickle frame that could be corrupted if the pressure was just right. As she had experienced earlier in life (she had a trauma history), people do not respect one another's space and can enter at will. She thus had never learned about healthy separateness. In my urge to "check off" one of our sessions because it was convenient for my schedule, I failed to reaffirm the necessary parameters of our relationship, even if doing so might have resulted in momentary anger and disappointment (which could have been my own imagining, as she had clearly stated she would leave and come back the next day). Rather, time was bent to accommodate her, giving her an uncomfortable omnipotence that reduced distance and limited frustration. Having too much access to those closest to her had always been tainted with a feeling of illicitness and guilt, given her early abuse. Her boundaries had been violated by those she trusted, closeness becoming associated with a confusing overstimulation. Any sense of omnipotence a child may have, even if developmentally appropriate, needs to be counterbalanced by a quota of frustration in order to maintain a sense of reality, to keep the fantasy from becoming too powerful and the child from having the terrible concern that there is no safety to be found, no boundaries to be had. It is necessary for caregivers to establish clear limits with a child and not allow the latter's impulses to be too consequential, because the child will not otherwise have the ability to process what is happening. When such limits are not in place, boundaries become fluid; intimacy is equated with intrusiveness and disorganization. While this form of relating might become a blueprint in the patient's life, it can be a devastating realization to have the therapist fall prey to such a traumatizing dynamic (even in subtle forms, as in the vignette) because the patient learns there is no safe harbor, and all seas are stormy. We may think it is inconsequential to "be flexible" for patients, but there is a deep dynamic meaning to *any* changes in the frame, and as in this example, our concrete changes can send shock waves through what is often the most predictable, reliable, and safe space in a patient's life.

Vignette 2

A highly intelligent Hungarian patient of mine was very preoccupied with my religious background. Specifically, he wanted to know if I was Catholic. When thinking about this in sessions, he was initially more playful and humorous when he approached the matter, not sticking with it much when I tried to understand why it was important to him. Over time, he became serious and much more fixated on the matter. I felt increasing pressure to give him a "yes" or "no" response. In fact, I wondered if doing so might actually free things up more because my "resistance" seemed to really stop up his associations, as he would stare at me with what I can only characterize as increasing bewilderment. My responses to him drew from the playbook in all the varieties with which I was familiar: "Let's think about the question together"; "What would it mean to you if I said 'yes,' and what would it mean if I said 'no'?"; "How do you feel about the fact that you haven't been able to get a straight answer from me?" Such incursions did little to allay his desire to know. I started to feel very uneasy before and during our sessions, as he became more impatient with my responses. We reached the point of having an entire session in which, from start to finish, *all* we spoke of was this. He threatened to stop coming to see me if I did not tell him if I was Catholic. In our work, it seemed to me that his need to know my religious background was less related to having me understand his inner world or belief system (he was more of a religious scholar and not an active practitioner). Rather, I experienced it as his needing to know I could be thrown off balance, that I would capitulate, which would account for his rising indignation at what he might have seen as my stubbornness. His early history was significant for a great deal of taunting from his siblings and even from his parents, given that several interests he cultivated were frowned upon by them. He enjoyed the arts and kept a journal of drawings, which at one point his father snatched from his hands and proceeded to show to everyone in the family, with people taking turns howling with laughter. It was profoundly shameful for him; his privacy and his right to keep his own interests in a "sacred" place beyond anyone else's reach were violated. He was forced to give up something concrete of his own, something important to him, something he would have rather kept hidden, to satisfy a forceful figure who did not respect the boundary. It was a terrible place for him to be in. Ultimately, I ran out of exploratory questions or statements. I voiced my bottom line. During one session, he said:

P: I want to know. Enough of this. Tell me right now: are you Catholic?
T: I'm not going to tell you.

His facial features progressed very quickly from what I interpreted as affronted astonishment, to anger, to resignation, to relieved humor.

P: Well, I guess that's that.
T (*sighing*): It's frustrating being with someone who has a mind of his own.

I believe this last statement on my part was as much a reflection of how I felt he was experiencing me as it was an acknowledgment of *my own* annoyance with the incessant questioning.

P: Yes, it is. I was never allowed that luxury. Let's move on.

Though initially frustrating, I thought this interaction conveyed that there were more benign ways of relating than one attempting a forced entry and the other helplessly submitting. I interpreted his reassured look as a realization that our dynamic would not be a reliving of aggressive attempts to expose one another at all costs. Rather, we could share our thoughts more quietly, respecting the limits we each needed to keep in place. The work proceeded very productively moving forward.

KEY POINTS

- The psychotherapeutic frame is sacred. It is a grounding presence that allows us to be available in ways that are predictable and reliable, though also limited.

- Through exploration of a patient's reactions to our intermittent availability, we can understand how our presence and absence resonate with their internal object relationships.

- Maintaining a consistent frame will further our ability to explore the meanings behind lateness, cancellations, and a patient's response to breaks in treatment (e.g., during vacations or holidays).

- Similarly, when the therapist impinges on or modifies the frame, this may be a recapitulation of a less reliable or sturdy object in a patient's life. This creates an opportunity to understand with our patients what may have been reenacted within our dyad.

References

Allen A: The fee as a therapeutic tool. Psychoanal Q 40(1):132–140, 1971 5100897

Auchincloss E, Samberg E: Psychoanalytic Terms and Concepts, 4th Edition. New Haven, CT, Yale University Press, 2012

Ferenczi S: Confusion of the tongues between the adults and the child—(the language of tenderness and of passion). Int J Psychoanal 30:225–230, 1949

Freud A: The ego and the mechanisms of defence, in The Writings of Anna Freud, Vol 2. New York, International Universities Press, 1936

Freud S: Lines of advance in psycho-analytic therapy (1919), in The Standard Edition of the Complete Psychological Works of Sigmund Freud, Vol 17. Translated and edited by Strachey J. London, Hogarth Press, 1955, pp 157–168

Furlong A: Some technical and theoretical considerations regarding the missed session. Int J Psychoanal 73 (Pt 4):701–718, 1992 1483849

Gabbard GO: What is a "good enough" termination? J Am Psychoanal Assoc 57(3):575–594, 2009 19620466

Greenson R: The Technique and Practice of Psychoanalysis, Vol 1. Madison, CT, International Universities Press, 1967

Joseph B: On understanding and not understanding: some technical issues. Int J Psychoanal 64 (Pt 3):291–298, 1983 6618778

Myers K: Show me the money: (the "problem" of) the therapist's desire, subjectivity, and relationship to the fee. Contemp Psychoanal 44:118–140, 2008

Pauley D: The therapeutics of the fee in psychoanalysis. Psychoanal Dialogues 29:560–574, 2019

Winnicott DW: Hate in the counter-transference. Int J Psychoanal 30:69–74, 1949

Words and Silence

Say little, do little, *that's my only salvation.*

Stendhal (1830/2008, p. 346;
emphasis in original)

[I]t is only in recent years that I have become able to wait and wait for the natural evolution of the transference arising out of the patient's growing trust in the psychoanalytic technique and setting, and to avoid breaking up this natural process by making interpretations.

Donald Winnicott (1969, p. 711)

ONE OF THE GREATEST challenges in becoming a therapist is being comfortable with silence. It may feel that unless someone is saying *something*, therapy is not taking place and time is being wasted. However, the use of silence as an *intervention* can be very effective and deepen the work. There is not always something to be said, and quiet reflection may be required to generate the next association. Patients sometimes stop and look at me in a session and pose the dilemma rather directly: "I don't know what to say next." I often respond simply, "Maybe nothing right now" or "Let's see what comes to mind next."

Similarly, during the course of a session, if the therapist makes an interpretation or a clarifying statement, we cannot expect immediate assimilation by the patient, nor a quickfire flow of subsequent associations. The same goes for therapists thinking about what patients say. Time is needed for words to be pondered, struggled with, associated to, and elaborated on. I certainly do not always have something to say after a patient speaks at some length and then grows quiet. If I cannot top silence, I say nothing. I can certainly appreciate the difficulty in remaining silent during high-tension moments with patients, as well as the push to rid myself of such unpleasantness by just saying *something*. However, to do so may be a strategy to address *my own* anxieties, using words as something concrete rather than symbolic, dislodging silence as opposed to communicating insight.

Returning to one of the principles of the object relations lens outlined in Chapter 1 ("Introduction")—"What is taking place in the room at this time between my patient and me?"—it is useful to think about how we notice ourselves interacting with specific patients, including a sense of urgency to speak versus the ability to be silent. With some patients, we have no problem sitting in silence, even for prolonged periods. With others, *any* moment of quietness is profoundly unsettling, as though the space created by silence needs to be immediately sewn up. The countertransference can help us learn something about our patients' inner worlds. (Indeed, a variant on the question posited earlier would be "What kind of object am I to this patient at this time?") Perhaps quiet curiosity was not something allowed by a patient's caregivers, who may have imposed their own presence and needs onto the child, demanding from the latter immediate and thoughtless responses. We may have had the experience of a patient talking at great length, followed immediately by our own interventions and back and forth, without an iota of silence. Yet we may leave such sessions with the feeling that *nothing* was actually communicated. Rather, a bunch of words were tossed about, and no further knowledge was acquired. In these instances, words are, in effect, used to keep real communication and understanding *out*. In such cases, the "insights" and viewpoints shared are ready-made, omniscience replacing doubt. Nothing can be left to chance because stopping could allow for an unexpected thought to arise, which might destabilize one's need to eliminate thinking by creating perennial static. Contrary to what Hamlet told Horatio, there are *not* more things in heaven and earth than have been dreamt of in one's philosophy.[1] It is helpful to catch ourselves when we are ready to jump in without having thought about why we are doing so, as though we are simply responding to a game of verbal "tag" in which we are now "it," and it is our turn to talk. The more we feel pulled to "do" something, the more we should refrain from doing *anything* until we can understand the pressures to which we are responding. So how might this play out on a practical level?

---

[1] Cf. Hamlet, I.v.168–169 (Shakespeare 1600/2016).

Cultivating Silence

I could understand the stillness in the house, and the thoughtfulness it expressed on the part of all those who had always been so good to me. I could weep in the exquisite felicity of my heart, and be as happy in my weakness as ever I had been in my strength.

Charles Dickens (1852–1853/1977, p. 432)

I am a big fan of allowing patients to start sessions. This avoids the "How are you?" or "Tell me about the week" snare, which may shunt the session in a direction our patients do not necessarily wish to go and move us away from something more immediately salient. I usually allow the patient to talk first, even if it takes a while. The world from which patients enter our offices is often one of incessant noise: the demands of work, school, partner, children, bills, and many others buzz about. The patient might *need* time to settle into the sessions. Silence becomes an ally to facilitate genuine communication. One might see the patient starting a session as akin to the caregiver allowing the child to express a gesture independently and then meeting the child's gesture. Beginning sessions in silence allows patients to start therapy on their own terms, without our prioritizing where *our* minds are as the way to begin the hour. If we agree with Zora Neale Hurston that the "oldest human longing" is self-revelation (Hurston 1937, p. 7), we need to be able to create a setting in which this can take place.

In therapy, there is much to learn from how patients reengage with us at the beginning of a new session. Their minds may be in strikingly different places since we last spoke, and they might wish to speak to something having *nothing* to do with where we left off last time or with any opening questions we may posit. Perhaps there was a lingering issue they did not address the previous week; they might have noticed something the very moment they walked in that did not seem quite right; maybe bits of a dream just came to mind as they saw us. It is a respect for the otherness and spontaneity of our patients' minds to allow them to reintroduce themselves to us as they see fit. If we are inviting a timelessness to the associative process, we should not rely on the passing of a certain number of seconds or minutes before one needs to break the silence.

In the film *Good Will Hunting* (1997), the title character (played by Matt Damon) is mandated to go to therapy. He mocks the process and alienates the therapists he sees. When he meets Sean (Robin Williams), he attempts to unnerve the latter as well and indeed manages to do so. Sean does not give up on him though but rather comes to appreciate the minefield he is entering by trying to make contact with this bright young man in his office. Will's traumatic past has alerted him to arm himself against anyone who approaches, shooting down any attempts to be reached. The only tactic Sean is left with is silence. An entire session goes by without either person saying a word; as this takes place, Will sits counting the seconds. On discussing the dynamic with a colleague, Sean sums up his position: "I can't talk first." When Will finally does decide to speak (as Sean is dozing off), he does so through a joke, neutralizing the battleground through playfulness. The therapist is now allowed in, and words can be used.

Sometimes residents tell me it feels off-putting to be silent at the beginning of a session. This is where psychoeducation becomes key. Rather than "just being silent" from the get-go without any grounding or contextualization as to why we are adopting this approach, patients should be told that they will be given the opportunity to start the sessions because this will open space for whatever is on their minds without the therapist directing things too much. Patients usually adjust to this pretty quickly, and the beginnings of sessions are quite fascinating if we allow them to unfold in such a manner. Of course, the therapist needs to meet patients where they are, and for some people, sitting in silence can feel intolerable. We adjust accordingly and may need to be more vocally present until the patient develops greater comfort with the dynamic. (Indeed, for some patients, perhaps the entire course of treatment will be marked by our speaking more than usual; this is not a failure but rather the dynamic that was found to be most helpful for *these particular individuals*, which is always the most important consideration.) We do not want to favor technique at all costs over building rapport, without which the most sophisticated technique is completely useless. Patients can feel very anxious about being met by a therapist's silence because it may suggest lack of concern, a judgmental stance, or any other number of possibilities. We try to make sense of patients and they try to make sense of us, but they are at a disadvantage given our nondisclosing stance. Just as their minds may not be in the same place between the end of one session and the beginning of the next, patients can never be sure they are coming back to the same therapist week after week. As such, they are often quite attuned to the "feel" of the session. A patient of mine would come into sessions and comment on the temperature of the room, in an uneasy way, and then proceed to ask me if *I* felt the same way. He was unsure if we shared the same atmosphere and if we could coexist in a harmonious manner. A supervisee, the day she decided to "start being psychodynamic" and not speak as much during sessions, noted the first thing her male patient said upon entering the room was that the pictures on the wall had switched places (which objectively was not true). There was *something* about the room this patient was walking into that was not the same. The therapist's mind was not the same, and perhaps it was *this* that was being registered on some level—he was picking up on a reality that was true to *him*. The object in the room with him was not the same.

Making small talk may serve to ground patients in the safety of the setting, with the "how are you?" and "nice weather" and the like possibly serving as encrypted forms of "please don't be mad at me for missing last time" or "I hope you still like me and will tolerate what I have to say." As mentioned, we want to be sensitive to what makes sense for each patient, and sometimes engaging in such small talk is necessary for some time to allow for a trusting alliance to develop. There is something sensory to the use of words that can provide warmth and welcoming. Whether we find ourselves talking or not, we should always think about what is taking place in the transference-countertransference as such dialogues are unfolding, with the hopes we will be able to take this up with the patient at some point, when things are more settled and words can be used differently. We should always strive to remain in a thinking place, whether we are speaking or in silence. It is through cultivating an open, soft stillness in our minds that we are better able to come in touch with what is alive in the here and now of the session, providing us the opportunity to understand what type of object we are to a patient in a given moment. As I tell trainees, we can always *think* psychodynamically about a patient, even if we cannot always *intervene* psychodynamically.

Whatever we say and whenever we choose to say it, a useful technical rule of thumb is that our intervention should be in the service of facilitating exploration, as opposed to shutting it down. Sometimes this will be through silence, speech, or simple body language; we need to be attentive to what the patient needs from us in the moment to move the process forward.

When there is a period of silence during a session, and after the patient resumes talking, I find it useful to ask what came to mind during the silence. This allows for a bridge to be created between the moment the patient stopped talking and when speech was resumed. (I have been quite surprised at how intricately patients can re-create their thought processes during those silent times, weaving through the numerous associations they had until the next vocalization was reached.)

I want to return to the concept that silence can be seen as an intervention just as valid as talking. Being quietly present with patients can be powerfully containing. I sometimes feel that I have said next to nothing over the course of 50 minutes (though feeling engaged and attentive the whole time) yet have been met with an amazing array of self-driven explorations, associations, and reflections, with the voiced statement at the end, "That was incredibly helpful. Thank you for listening." Far from the feeling one sometimes has that words are being used as a mechanical force to push out the therapist and any ability to think more deeply, these types of sessions are examples of patients being able to "play in the presence of the other" (i.e., exploration is allowed and encouraged by the quiet, actively listening therapist). Our words are often less important than our working and attentive minds, and it may very well feel (to echo the statement by Winnicott from the beginning of this chapter) that to interpret would actually *interfere* with insight rather than promote it.

The Therapist Speaks

We do, of course, need to speak at some point. Although silence is golden, there is a balance that must be struck between quietly allowing for patients to feel at ease within sessions without imposing our own mental content and speaking to their experience in a way that can deepen the work and facilitate exploration. Too *much* silence can be part of an enactment, too, and we may be experienced over time as someone who cannot make sense of the patient's inner world, with the therapist's silence evoking a feeling of despair as opposed to containment. We do have working minds, and these minds are rarely quiet. It is *how* we share our thoughts with patients that is instrumental.

As we try to find a way to communicate our understanding or lack thereof, there are infinite choices to draw from. Nodding or gently acquiescing with a "yes" or "uh-huh" may be radically different from maintaining a warmly attentive gaze and making statements such as "huh" or "hmm." In his book on psychoanalytic technique, Lacanian psychoanalyst Bruce Fink suggests developing a whole repertoire of noises to be uttered in response to what patients say (Fink 2007). He outlines the difference between saying something like "hmm" versus "uh-huh." While the former is a recognition that the patient said something and that the therapist is present and listening, the latter contains within it something of an implicit acknowledgment that what the patient said was understood. Even a simple mental exercise of imagining ourselves saying something to someone and being received with one utterance versus the other will allow us to conjure the impact each response would have on us and what we might think is going on in the mind of the listener. "Hmm" can be seen as a statement of presence but not of commitment, opening space for the patient's associations to our response. I can certainly appreciate the pressures to say something that is superficially more reassuring but also realize it may mislead my patients into thinking I know exactly what they are talking about, when this may be far from true. In my fledgling therapist days, I experimented with these different technical approaches and found that trying to remain in a space of noncommittal openness (whether through more neutral statements or by catching myself so I did not nod too much in agreement) helped with *my own* sense of grounding. It also allows for whatever projective pressures are in the room to come to the fore, and the work can deepen without our having to do much other than allow stillness. In a way, a patient who is vigilant about surface indicators of reassurance or immediate understanding might be very worried about what may happen if these indicators are not visible at all times.

Even if we feel we *do* understand what a patient is saying in a given moment, we should give due consideration to the trickiness of language. It is a tenuous proposition to say that we "get" what patients are telling us or that the descriptors used for their emotional states allow for an accurate evocation in our minds of how they are subjectively feeling (e.g., we just "know" what they mean when they tell us they are angry, scared, or sad). Language, in effect, is a limited and distorted form of relaying one's internal experiences. Freud contended that the ego is, first and foremost, a body-ego (Freud 1923/1961, p. 27). The earliest forms of containment in the caregiver-infant dyad predate verbal and symbolic communication, taking place on a level of autonomic modulation, with soothing being predicated on an attunement that does not rely on vocabulary but on a physical, sensorial presence. As we emerge from a sensorimotor world into one in which communication becomes increasingly verbal, the use of words will be turned to as a means of describing impossibly complex body states and emotional processes, which until then were simply lived out. As richly complex as a vocabulary may be, it is insufficient to convey the depth and scope of human experience, which is never stagnant and is arguably ineffable in its essence. We can look at verbal communication between two individuals as somewhat akin to an hourglass (Figure 4–1). In the center, or neck, of the hourglass, one can imagine a statement—for instance, "I'm angry."

If we turn the hourglass on its side, there are two expanses emanating from the neck, in opposite directions. One expanse represents the patient's perspective, informed by life history and individual subjectivity, and the other expanse represents the perspective of the therapist, whose *own* subjectivity will be drawn from when associating to the word in question. These two subjective worlds converge at that middle point, where words are used as a means of bringing something from one person's inner world to the awareness of the listener. As such, the patient's expanse or experience will find its voice in the word *angry*. Upon hearing this word, the therapist's expanse or experience will be activated, with individual associations coming to mind that may be significantly different from the ones the patient wished to convey. It is highly improbable (and perhaps even strike the reader as impossible) that these two expanses could ever entirely coincide. However, as improbable as it seems, the existence of such an overlap is implied to patients when they say "I'm angry" and we say "I understand." It is a potentially problematic re-

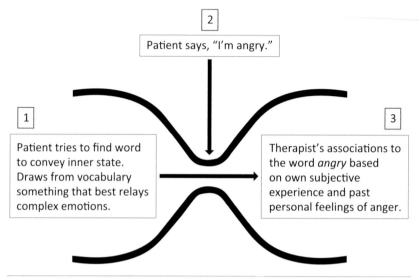

Figure 4–1.   Convergence and divergence in attempting to
              communicate inner experience.

sponse on our part because we are making quite a leap in saying that. I have found that simply repeating the word back suspends it between the two of us, giving it room to breathe and be unpacked without its being hastily assigned meaning. The therapist says "Angry" and waits to see what happens next. The patient may (and usually does) spontaneously elaborate, having been given permission to delve deeper. This can be quite encouraging for patients because they might be struggling to find the words, and premature "understanding" by the therapist closes down the need to wrestle with this word and its implications before laying it to rest as a statement of crystal-clear connotations.[2]

Alternatively, there might be an expectation that the therapist should know *exactly* what the meaning of this word is—"Yeah, *angry*. You know what

---

[2] In *Philosophical Investigations*, Ludwig Wittgenstein (1953/2009) proposed the thought experiment in which several people would be together, each person holding an individual box and claiming that inside the box was a "beetle." However, no one could look into the other's box, so no one could ever really know if the object that one person was calling a beetle was the same as the object in the other person's box, also called a beetle. He went on to say, "Here it would be quite possible for everyone to have something different in his box. One might even imagine such a thing constantly changing(...)the box might even be empty" (1.293; p. 106ᵉ).

that is, don't you?" Now, this feels like a fork-in-the-road scenario, which can play out in different ways. Perhaps the therapist, suddenly feeling exposed and clumsy, will try to adhere to the patient in a way that eliminates tension and difference between the two. For instance, if a patient was raised by an oppressive and authoritarian caregiver, we can imagine an internalized object relationship in which one individual is placing strong demands on the other, with no regard for how scared and exposed the latter might feel. As a child, the patient might have felt quite intimidated and under pressure to conform to the views and requirements of the powerful authority figure. When we are suddenly being pressured to say we understand what the patient is saying, even though we really do *not*, we find ourselves in the very same situation the patient was in during that earlier stage in life. This would be an instance of projective identification, wherein we feel pressured to *relive this particular form of relating* the patient internalized from the past. Importantly, in projective identification, we may be assigned either role within the object relationship—that is, taking on the characteristics of an early figure or of the patients themselves. In the latter case, we understand on a visceral level the pressures *the patient* faced when a caregiver or important other was making demands for understanding to occur when the cognitive wherewithal to do so simply was not there. Through this "turning passive into active," the patient takes on the role of intolerant adult, placing impossible demands on someone without providing that person with the necessary tools to complete such a task. The patient does not wish to be caught needing to explain what is meant by the choice of this word; something about it feels too distressing and exposing (indeed, the therapist's repeating the word back might feel like an indictment that the patient is not being clear or is doing therapy incorrectly). Through projective identification, the tables are turned, and the pressures are placed on *us*. The therapist might quickly say, "Oh yes, angry—I do understand, of course." Neither party is exposed anymore, and the enactment is completed without any further thought to it. Yet the anxieties residing beneath the surface are intact. The patient, once again, is not understood.

Taking a step back in such situations is not easy, but it is part and parcel of understanding the process occurring within the therapist-patient dyad at any given moment. In this particular example, the therapist, noticing the pressure mounting, can simply comment on this very situation. Owning the role (as opposed to pushing it away) helps speak to the active object relationship being repeated, reflecting on how this situation needed to play out as it did and what the threat would be were it to proceed differently. The therapist could say, "It sounds like I messed up by not knowing exactly what you meant by 'angry'" (indicating the patient was in the role of one making such a demand and the therapist was the inept individual failing to meet expectations—i.e., the therapist is in the role of patient-as-child) or "If I just assumed I *knew* what you meant based on my *own* definition of 'anger,' what you actually hoped to communicate through that word is dropped and becomes lost" (as the patient was forced to conform to the caregiver's perspectives and opinions, in detriment of the patient's own internal experiences—i.e., the therapist is in the role of authoritarian caregiver).[3] Thus, a discussion can be fostered about how a past object relationship template is trying to find its way into the here and now, creating an opportunity for it to be understood instead of being blindly reenacted.

Creating space for something as minute as a single word to acquire such dimensionality requires taking one's foot off the mental accelerator. We need to keep ourselves in a relaxed and receptive place, yielding to the knowledge that a patient's mind can *never* be fully understood, and even when we *do* grasp something of the patient's experience, it is ephemeral because the mind can quickly move to being somewhere else. Giving ourselves permission to entertain grayness in such a way can, to borrow from Bion, "ease problems of thinking about something that is unknown" (Bion 1962, p. 89). The mind can go anywhere if given the chance. Cognizance of the ever-evolving nature of the human psyche allows us to welcome its untamed ways. We become fascinated by it and want to play with it. We recognize our inability to ever keep up with its awesome prowess. As Winnicott (1969) stated, "I think I interpret mainly to let the patient know the limits of my understanding" (p. 711).

Questions Versus Statements

One other technical recommendation I make is that if the therapist has a query in mind during a session, one should try to find a way of formulating it into a statement, as opposed to asking the question. This takes some pres-

---

[3] Cf. Heinrich Racker's (1957) distinction between concordant countertransference—in which the therapist identifies with dimensions of the patient's self-representation—and complementary countertransference—in which the therapist identifies with a patient's internal objects or object-representation. Racker characterized concordant countertransference as that in which the "intention to understand creates a certain predisposition, a predisposition to identify oneself with the analysand, which is the basis of comprehension. The analyst may achieve this aim by identifying his ego with the patient's ego or, to put it more clearly although with a certain terminological inexactitude, by identifying each part of his personality with the corresponding psychological part in the patient—his id with the patient's id, his ego with the ego, his superego with the superego, accepting these identifications in his consciousness" (p. 311). Regarding complementary countertransference, Racker stated that "the patient treats the analyst as an internal (projected) object, and in consequence the analyst feels treated as such" (p. 312).

sure off the patient because a question in essence demands an answer, and the time spent actually pondering the therapist's words might be lessened by feeling some urgency to respond. If the therapist asks, "How are you feeling?" the dynamic in the room is tilted in the direction of the patient, whose shoulders are now carrying the weight of having been asked something for which there is the expectation of a response. The therapist, in effect, is relieved of this pressure, in a way disenthralled of co-constructing the narrative of the session. This can feel unsettling, and a patient who is questioned might (as highlighted earlier) reproject this discomfort onto the therapist—"How do you *think* I'm feeling?" or "How are *you* feeling? Let's see how you like being hammered with questions." Another appealing aspect to making statements is that it draws us in more closely, making the therapist an active participant in the session. There is *always* an active object relationship in the room. We are there with our patients, and our interventions should reflect this. Though the difference may feel very subtle, in saying something like "I can see this has impacted you" or "I'm here thinking about how that must have felt for you," we are positioning ourselves a little differently, as someone with a thinking mind, with an individual presence, who is actively engaged with our patients in trying to make sense of their experience, without shifting the pressure too much onto them. When we make a statement, we are taking some ownership for our part in the relationship.[4] My observation is "sitting there." The patient can choose to take it up, think about it, drop it, or ignore it. In any event, we will have something to discuss.[5]

For some patients, there is a difficulty in *coming up* with their own words to characterize their internal state, leading to nebulous, circuitous descriptions that seem to circle around something more definitive without ever hitting it. In such instances, the therapist offering up a word that might help

---

[4] At some Kleinian discussion groups, when a therapist presents clinical material, often the rule is that participants are *not allowed* to ask questions. Rather, they need to make statements, sharing their reactions and making themselves active participants in the case. This makes for a discussion that feels more collective compared with dynamics in which the listeners ask question after question, which can feel very exposing for the presenter and safer for the questioners.

[5] This recommendation is, of course, one of several ways to approach sessions and is meant to help the therapist position oneself as an active object in the room. It is not always easy to configure one's thoughts into statements in the immediacy of an exchange, and indeed readers will notice that several vignettes in this book have questions posed by the therapist. This is not meant to be all or none, and therapists need to adopt the communicative style they feel best suits them. It can, however, be a useful experiment for trainees to try out in sessions, gauging how it feels to ask a question versus make a statement. Over time, I have opted increasingly for the latter and have felt much more actively co-participatory in sessions with my patients.

add some verbal grounding to the emotion can be useful—"I wonder if you felt angry" or "Sounds like a distressing experience." The purpose is the same as the earlier observations (i.e., when a patient names an emotion and we ponder the word's significance)—it is meant to find a way to further access the patient's subjectivity. Even if the patient agrees—"Yes, I was angry"—this is a nodal point that does not stop associations but invites further ones: the therapist can say, "Tell me more." If we name the emotion, it is not an all-encompassing, explanatory intervention on our part. Rather, it is an invitation for patients to sit with the idea, think about it, and contrast their own thoughts against it. If we say something like "I think you're upset with me," the patient may feel encouraged to say, "No, that's not quite it," and engage in a process of discussion around something that, although maybe not exactly right, has helped provide material for a joint thinking process, working together to give shape to something that might have felt much more formless. Other times, we may be spot-on, the patient feeling relieved that we have been able to help find a way to speak about something that seemed out of reach or off limits; it is suddenly plainly present and available for discussion. Such a contribution is a summoning from the therapist's internal world, requiring a *dialogue* with that of the patient rather than subsuming or replacing it. It is a statement of our momentary sense of what we are hearing, with all the inherent limitations carried by our point of view. It is a statement of our presence inviting the reaction of our dyadic co-constructor.

As an important aside—when we do speak, whatever we are saying, however we are saying it (whether question or statement or other), our contributions should be stated *in plain words*, as opposed to being oracular or attempting some deep, all-encompassing interpretation. Speaking in a relatable way bridges the chasm between therapist and patient; it represents the search for a form of communication that can be grasped by *both*, bringing the two closer to a shared truth.

Along these lines, I also encourage residents not to use abstract words when referring to themselves in the sessions. It is not uncommon for therapists to speak of themselves as some disembodied figure in the room, with phrases such as "Do you think the therapy is contributing to this?" or "How does this apply to your therapist?" being quite common. We may speak as though we were not allowed to be real humans in the room. This can be a protective (albeit defensive) way of removing ourselves from the intensity of session dynamics, adopting the alienating cloak of "the therapist." I encourage residents to use the *I* and *me* pronouns when referring to themselves. If I want to think about the sessions through the lens of an object relationship, my language needs to reflect my role as an active participant.

Clinical Vignette

A woman I worked with in therapy tried to interest me in her business ventures. With great animation, she told me that her primary care physician was ready to invest in the promising stock options she told him about. She had a history of going bankrupt some years prior after her ex-husband invested their money recklessly. I appreciated her need to move away from that devastating reality and the pain that revisiting it in session might lead to. By turning to a "manic" solution to the situation (see Chapter 8, "The Oedipal Situation [Exclusion and Rivalry]: Theory"), she was jumping inside my mind and trying to draw me into the excitement of resolving conflict through immediate action. In joining her, I would be losing my own footing as a therapist and bankrupting my thinking abilities.

> P: It's a wonderful opportunity. My primary doctor knows all about it. He's in. He invested thousands already. I'll give you the information, and you can invest, too.
> T: You're telling me *anyone* would find it too tempting to pass up.
> P: It *is*! I'm digging my way out of the hole. You in?

Incidentally, this was happening at the tail end of the session (with a couple of minutes remaining), and the patient was already gathering her things to leave. It was an inversion of the more familiar end-of-session dynamic, wherein the patient has to leave despite perhaps wanting more from the therapist. In this case, she was creating a scenario in which *I* would want more from *her*, and I had to decide if I was going to take it before it was too late. I was trying to remain in a thinking place, wondering how I could find some grounding when both our minds were under such pressure to merge into something frantic and unthinking. I went with the only thing that sprang to mind in the moment.

> T: Hmm…
> P: [Stops packing up her things and stares intently at me.] "Hmm" *what*? What does that noise even *mean*?
> T: Your thoughts? [I'm becoming anxious.]
> P: *My* thoughts? I'm telling *you* about something that could help *you*! My other doctor wasn't like this.
> T: [More anxiety] You may be upset that I'm making the therapy about how *I* might help *you*, as opposed to being drawn into the excitement of how both our lives could be fixed without any of this therapy stuff being necessary.
> P: You're killing my high….I don't like that. Fine, never mind. My ex-husband wasn't like this.

My "Hmm" was the only intervention I could muster to weather the storm. It was a sound of presence, an unformulated reaction to the circumstances, and a reflection of my inability to say anything else. It was sufficient to evoke a strong response from the patient, literally halting all activity (both verbally and behaviorally, as she stopped packing to stare) and allowing for further associations to be generated. I became a different type of object for her, one that prioritized thinking together instead of acting together—in stark contrast to the mindset shown by her ex-husband and primary doctor, as she pointed out. At times, such simple interventions can deepen the process more than fancy explanations or theorizing. (In the vignette, I think the "Hmm" was more effective in creating space for exploration than any of my other comments.)

Sitting with our anxiety and resisting the pull to reenact is not easy. (It can be downright miserable.) Through projective identification, the therapist is pressured *"to live out a part of the patient's self instead of analysing it"* (Joseph 1975/1989, p. 86; emphasis in original). Because my patient could not tolerate the notion that her venture could be ill-fated, all the potentially negative aspects were split off and eliminated from her mind. Lest I be seen as the party pooper, a container for these ejected, unwelcome bits of reality, I experienced the push to comply and join in the excitement, though this would require sacrificing my own thinking mind in the process. As Feldman (1999) mentioned, "The disturbing phantasy (or reality) for the analyst is that when he resists the pressure for such compliance, he has to tolerate the anxiety, discomfort, and guilt associated with being the cruel, sadistic, spoiling person" (p. 33).

When we maintain our ground, not agreeing with the idea that "there is nothing more to see here," we risk being seen as a confusing and persecutory object; it is akin to dragging someone to the hangover state before the intoxication has been enjoyed. Yet it is our role to keep these unpleasant aspects in mind as we work with patients, while understanding and empathizing with the latter's need to jettison them because they may conjure up a tremendous amount of pain.

KEY POINTS

- Silence can be a powerful intervention in sessions. The therapist needs to find a balance between when to remain quietly receptive and when to be vocally active.

- Fundamentally, it is crucial for the therapist to remain in a grounded, thinking place in order to understand and speak to the projective pressures in the room.

- Often, we may find ourselves speaking to "fill the air," with little communicative function behind our speech. It is important to notice when words are being used (by the therapist, patient, or both) to deepen the exploratory process and when they are used to stifle it.

References

Bion W: Learning From Experience. London, Karnac, 1962

Dickens C: Bleak House (1852–1853). Norton Critical Edition. New York, WW Norton, 1977

Feldman M: The defensive uses of compliance. Psychoanal Inq 19:22–39, 1999

Fink B: Fundamentals of Psychoanalytic Technique: A Lacanian Approach for Practitioners. New York, WW Norton, 2007

Freud S: The ego and the id (1923), in The Standard Edition of the Complete Psychological Works of Sigmund Freud, Vol 19. Translated and edited by Strachey J. London, Hogarth Press, 1961, pp 1–66

Hurston ZN: Their Eyes Were Watching God. New York, HarperCollins, 1937

Joseph B: The patient who is difficult to reach (1975), in Psychic Equilibrium and Psychic Change: Selected Papers of Betty Joseph. Edited by Feldman M, Spillius EB. New York, Routledge, 1989, pp 75–87

Racker H: The meanings and uses of countertransference. Psychoanal Q 26:303–357, 1957 13465913

Shakespeare W: Hamlet (1600). : The Pelican Shakespeare. New York, Penguin Books, 2016

Stendhal: The Red and the Black (1830). Norton Critical Edition. New York, WW Norton, 2008

Winnicott DW: The use of an object. Int J Psychoanal 50:711–716, 1969

Wittgenstein L: Philosophical Investigations (1953). Chichester, West Sussex, UK, Wiley-Blackwell, 2009

Finding the Focus:
Content Versus Process

*He that has eyes to see and ears to hear may convince himself that
no mortal can keep a secret. If his lips are silent, he chatters with his
finger-tips; betrayal oozes out of him at every pore. And thus the
task of making conscious the most hidden recesses of the mind is one
which it is quite possible to accomplish.*

Sigmund Freud (1905[1901]/1953, pp. 77–78)

*[O]ne of the most effective interventions with my patients is not
what I am doing, but how I am being.*

Richard Chefetz (2017, p. 122)

WHAT WE SAY is sometimes not as important as *how* we say it. Intonation,
volume, stressing particular syllables, and body language are crucial aspects
of communication, elevating the power and nuance of speech beyond the
combination of words composing it. Also, the state of mind a person is in
when listening to something will influence its meaning and impact. The
same stimulus may not be experienced the same way at different times because our emotions play a role in filtering it. Imagine receiving a phone call
or text message; without seeing who the caller or texter is, we will assign a
particular meaning to it depending on how we are feeling. We might be very
open to receiving a message from someone or in the mood for engaging in
lively conversation; in such an instance, that little noise may bring us some
excitement and expectation. At other times, we might be in a foul, withdrawn, and miserable mood, unwelcoming of *any* human contact. Hearing

the grating noise of the phone going off might make us want to smash it against the wall. Same noise, different response. This is a rather simplistic but useful example of what a "process" versus "content" consideration may entail. The noise from the phone is the *content* it is producing. The *process* is the greater context in which content is being delivered; this context includes a great deal of subjectivity (as in the example), further complicating matters when there is more than one person involved.

The "Process" of Saying Things

In psychotherapy, what the patient is saying, the words themselves, can be viewed as "content." Content is tremendously important because it gives us an idea of what is on the patient's mind consciously and (indirectly) provides insights into the workings of the unconscious, as buried memories arise, dreams are shared, and slips of the tongue are pondered. However, we must always think about the greater context in which content is being expressed (Isaacs 1948). There is a powerful nonverbal communication ("action language") that runs parallel to the verbal exchange in a session. The experiential domain of the encounter is punctuated by the affective tone; the nondescript "feel" of the room, conferring a sense of safety or threat; and the interpersonal rhythm the dyad maintains in times of silence and when conversing. All of these dimensions constitute the very essence of an object relationship being lived in the here and now.

What *is* the process in psychotherapy? It can be defined, maybe oversimplistically, as how a patient communicates with us in a session, as opposed to what is being stated. A feeling of trust and safety in a session can allow for a patient to speak more freely, deepening associations through a joint processing. We notice, in such instances, an open body language, relaxed (and even excited) facial expressions, and a process of delivering speech that is harmonious with the deepening of content. Very differently, a patient's body language might be closed off, with gloomy or disengaged facial expressions and a gaze that is constantly avoiding that of the therapist. The "emotional temperature" in the room might be one of disconcerting coldness. Irrespective of *what* a patient says in such a situation, it needs to be thought about against this backdrop of possible mistrust or wariness.

When content is not being used to facilitate actual communication, sessions might be marked by a lot of words or by silence (as well as by remarkable combinations of the two). We may feel invaded by ceaseless chatter, unable to keep up with the labyrinthine associations, name-dropping of people we have never met, and long stretches of accelerated speech. This can cause us to feel overwhelmed and pushed out, unable to think, write, or contribute in any meaningful way. When the patient *does* stop talking, many times this is accompanied by a stare, a nonverbal "it's your turn to talk, so hurry up" nudge, which can be *very* difficult to sit with. Often, when faced with such a dynamic, we *do* end up saying something trite and unhelpful, maybe even a useless "clarifying" question, which does nothing other than cue the patient to launch into another tornado of words. Patients may be very worried about what might happen were there to be silence in the session. If the therapist and the patient can quietly access their respective minds, something unexpected might emerge, causing a disruption from which the patient might not know how to recover. When thinking needs to be avoided, psychological mindedness is something to be defended against.[1] In such a situation, we need not think as much about *what* is being said to us but rather *how* words are being used to keep us out.

In other situations, patients might be largely withdrawn, remaining silent for extended periods of time, sometimes for entire sessions. It might feel that patients are refusing to give us the satisfaction of engaging with psychotherapy, viewing their words as currency—if they speak, they impoverish themselves and make us richer and more powerful. Other patients carefully measure and edit their words to "ensure" there is no danger of the therapist's mind misconstruing meaning. After something is said, it is no longer under the control of the speaker. The mind of the other can be a frightening thing indeed, and its potential to cause damage through its own thinking process is a common anxiety for patients. One female patient caught herself in the middle of a sentence—"Whenever it's time for our session and you come to pick me up…I mean, *get* me, I start to think about the first thing I'll say to you when we begin." I observed that she had changed her language midsentence. She said, "Yeah, it's a little embarrassing. I didn't want you to misunderstand me, that I was saying you were going to pick me up, like on a date. That's *not* what I meant at all." It is notable that the possibility of such a (mis)construal was attributed to *me*, through a quickfire projection—the idea of an erotic dimension to our relationship was generated in *her* mind, led to discomfort, became *my* issue, and was then neutralized by a change in the content of the speech. It has been floated about in psychodynamic theory that there is no negative in the unconscious and that if a patient uses the word *not* (or its variants) in a sentence, we should pretend the word is absent if we wish to come closer to the truth. If someone says, "Why, I absolutely do *not* want to kill my brother!" we can see how the sentence becomes problematic if we remove *not*. Some wishes are too overwhelming for patients' psyches; it is only by denying the idea entirely, turning it into its opposite, or locating it in others (through

---

[1] *Psychological mindedness* refers to the awareness that unknown or unconscious factors may play a role in shaping conflicts and symptoms.

projection) that it can be made available for conscious processing.[2] Once the idea is on the table, it can be talked about. In the case of projection, it may be helpful to allow the attribute to stick with us a little bit (e.g., "You imagine *I* might have thought of picking you up on a date if you hadn't changed your words"), helping to detoxify an idea that felt *so* anxiety-provoking it needed to be pushed into the therapist. This might help a patient reclaim the thought as one's own, opening space for a discussion of why it felt so dangerous.

The state of mind patients are in will influence how they speak. Words are the gatekeepers of the mind, inviting or repudiating understanding, clarifying matters or fogging them up. In sessions, who *we* are for patients at any given time can change drastically. We may have a patient who comes into sessions with a subdued, resigned look, barely enunciating words and making minimal eye contact. During the interactions, we might find ourselves becoming angry, wanting to tell the patient to take the therapy seriously or else find a different provider. Even if the therapist does not make such egregious statements, the patient may sense tension in the room and notice a curtness in the therapist's responses. Feeling incompetent and forlorn, the patient may withdraw further and apologize for wasting the therapist's time. A different patient might engage with us in more openly critical ways, haughtily dismissing everything we say as "stupid" and "pointless," saying we have no business being therapists and that we had better step up our game or we would be left for someone "more qualified" who "isn't just a trainee." We come to feel terribly inept and start to question our chosen vocation. In these two contrasting scenarios, words are withheld or fired out in ways that cause us to experience opposite emotions—demanding or deprived, entitled or devalued. The *feel* in the room, the process taking place between therapist and patient, is much more salient than any actual content that was spoken (particularly in the first case, punctuated as it was by silence). Indeed, sometimes *nothing* is said, yet something powerful is felt. Even when patients are lying on the couch in psychoanalytic therapy, I can sense when they are tearing up, though they may not be speaking, and I am unable to see their faces. Our ability to relay our emotional state in such visceral ways underlines a dimension to human connectedness that transcends the most sophisticated use of speech. We

---

[2] This is in line with the idea that the id is a realm of the psyche in which everything is permitted; there is no time, no boundary, no limit; such permissiveness is contrary to the brakes that the concept of "no" would put into place. In his work titled "Negation," Freud (1925/1961) reiterated this: "In analysis we never discover a 'no' in the unconscious and that recognition of the unconscious on the part of the ego is expressed in a negative formula. There is no stronger evidence that we have been successful in our effort to uncover the unconscious than when the patient reacts to it with the words 'I didn't think that,' or 'I didn't (ever) think of that'" (p. 239).

might walk into a room with a patient and feel uneasy, hyperaware, and confused before *anything* has been said.

Despite words being the stock-in-trade in psychotherapy, there is much to be "said" about the nonverbal communication that is always taking place. Truths can be expressed through our pores, as the opening quote of this chapter suggests. This is a point argued by some who advocate for face-to-face psychotherapy because there is something irreplaceably informative about maintaining visual contact. This could be conceptualized as somewhat akin to early child-caregiver attunement dynamics, wherein communication is powerfully driven by visual exchange (Stern et al. 1998). Although the use of the couch in psychoanalysis has been kept in practice and can serve as a helpful tool for some patients, its historical roots are less than scientifically sound; the practice may have even derived from a need to move *away* from the intensity of maintaining eye contact during sessions. Freud (1913/1958) stated,

> I must say a word about a certain ceremonial which concerns the position in which the treatment is carried out. I hold to the plan of getting the patient to lie on a sofa while I sit behind him out of his sight. This arrangement has a historical basis; it is the remnant of the hypnotic method out of which psycho-analysis was evolved. But it deserves to be maintained for many reasons. The first is a personal motive, but one which others may share with me. I cannot put up with being stared at by other people for eight hours a day (or more). Since, while I am listening to the patient, I, too, give myself over to the current of my unconscious thoughts, I do not wish my expressions of face to give the patient material for interpretations or to influence him in what he tells me. (pp. 133–134)

Paying attention to the process helps us understand the type of object we are to patients at any given moment—how they are experiencing us can facilitate or inhibit the tide of their associations.[3] It is common for patients to come into a therapy session and say, "I had a very clear idea of what I wanted to say to you, but as soon as I walked into this office, it evaporated. I can't, for the life of me, remember anything." Mental content may be more accessible to consciousness when there is less danger of it being exposed, particularly if it is very anxiety-provoking or disturbing. Sharing this content with

---

[3] This is relevant for how patients respond to our interventions as well. In a sense, what we say may be less important than what the patient *does* with what we say. Varying responses can occur, depending on how we are being viewed. If we are experienced as a bad object, our most eloquent and insightful statements can fall flat; conversely, our clumsy and inarticulate comments may be gently held and sounded for meaning by a patient who is viewing us as a good object.

a therapist can be all the more challenging because the provider is likely to take the patient's words seriously and try to explore the matter further. One patient told me that he remembered his dreams quite vividly, even journaling them with an incredible level of detail. Then, when we started therapy, he started forgetting his dreams, even though he knew his mind was still producing them. He said this was probably because his dreams were very disturbing, and he had trouble imagining having a conversation about them, worrying I would "think he was crazy." The idea of revealing them to me might have caused danger alerts to go off in his unconscious mind. This hypothesis was furthered by the fact that during a 2-week vacation I took, he was suddenly able to remember his dreams just as vividly as before we started treatment.

If communication is truncated or openly attacked in sessions, we should try to think about this as a reliving of an internalized object relationship. After all, no matter how unhealthy certain dynamics might seem in sessions, patients are doing therapy the way that makes sense to them, and we need to be respectful of this. If sessions with a given patient are marked by feelings of unease, the therapist's inability to keep a straight thought, an empty tossing about of words by both individuals in the room, and an overall sense of stagnation and futility in treatment, we might wonder if some internalized template is repeating itself. In this template, communicating with another person does not lead to further understanding or psychic growth; rather, it results in a spinning of verbal wheels with no forward movement. As our frustrations mount, we may despair at this seemingly insoluble dynamic. However, I would suggest that we are *experientially* learning about the patient's past in ways to which objective descriptions could never do justice; we are *feeling* the past come to life in the present (Bergstein 2020). Critically, we might notice small movements in sessions: a smile, an uncrossing of the arms, some eye contact, or a brief increase in speech production. These moments may be followed by an almost immediate shutting down, but the word *almost* becomes instrumental because we have just witnessed the patient's potential for contact, for relatedness, and for some other way of being with us beyond the constraints of early object relationship models. Noticing these shifts in sessions can facilitate a discussion of what allowed the patient to feel more open (even if momentarily) and what pressures led to a closing off. This consideration will be expanded on later in this book (see Chapters 7, 8, and 9).

Continuity Across Sessions

When we are thinking about process as an evolving narrative, it is useful to remember that the work of therapy actively continues between sessions. After all, our patients will 1) have had *some* reaction to how the last session proceeded and ended, 2) have potentially furthered their introspection on the matters discussed, and 3) be in a particular state of mind upon returning for the next session. The process in place at the end of a session may be the result of an arduous effort by both members of the dyad to maintain an exploratory mindset; patients might be feeling safe and connected with the therapist when "minute 50" hits. It is time to stop. This is not easy because patients now need to return to a world that treats them very differently compared with the one they were just in. In the fast-paced and competitive society we live in, staying in a place of vulnerability is hardly compatible with a functional lifestyle. As such, defenses are mustered and walls constructed. What has been set in motion during the session—while it will continue to be active in the patient's subsequent thoughts, feelings, and dreams—cannot be expressed in the same way outside. It is not realistic to go around saying anything that comes to mind to everyone we meet and expect people to be open and curious about what we are saying. (The oft-used term *TMI* [too much information] is the social reminder of how unwelcome what we have to say really is.)

This potential for a patient's defenses to be strongly summoned between sessions underlines the need for encounters to be frequent enough to keep an exploratory process afloat, without prolonged interruptions. Regular, frequent appointments also allow for transference dynamics to be better understood because the therapist will become a more central figure for the patient. Freud (1913/1958) had an even more regimented way of working with patients. He stated,

> I work with my patients every day except on Sundays and public holidays—that is, as a rule, six days a week. For slight cases or the continuation of a treatment which is already well advanced, three days a week will be enough. (…) Even short interruptions have a slightly obscuring effect on the work. We used to speak jokingly of the "Monday crust" when we began work again after the rest on Sunday. (p. 127)

While we want to be cognizant of how the last session ended, patients are often in a *very* different place when returning to see us. We need to be open and receptive to this, remembering that our patients' minds have been very active since we last met. This is one reason why it can be very useful to allow patients to speak first in sessions (as discussed in Chapter 4, "Words and Silence"). One is reminded of Bion's controversial and oft-misunderstood statement that we should impose on ourselves the "positive discipline of eschewing memory and desire" (Bion 1970/2004, p. 31), suggesting we should not let the content covered in the previous session(s) overly occupy our minds when we meet our patients again, nor should we be burdened by our own "desire" for how patients should be living their lives or progressing clinically.[4]

A patient of mine would tell me I needed to keep good notes and be sure to hold her accountable for "picking up where [she] left off" from one session to the next because she did not wish to "waste time" by starting sessions with surface-level material before "getting to the important stuff." Notably, she struggled to start sessions on her own, giving me "the cue" to guide her through what I had written down. When she was met with silence, it was somewhat disconcerting, but she would eventually begin talking, rather thoughtfully, about matters either related to or completely different from where we had stopped the last time. The spontaneity and introspection she showed betrayed the reductionistic, "scripted" formula she had laid out for us. In effect, we were being set up for a reenactment. If I followed her oft-suggested technique of forcing her to "pick up where we left off," I would be showing no concern for where her mind might be from one moment (or session) to the next, as though her thoughts were something as two-dimensional and unchanging as whatever notes I had jotted down. After I presented this idea to her, she accessed a memory of her parents' quasi-draconian focus on grades and academic achievements, saying they would refer to periods in her life in relation to her performance at the time (e.g., "your soccer trophy May," "that June you got a B in history"). Anything taking place beyond these objective markers was dismissed as unimportant. I was being invited to play a similar role with her, guiding the direction of sessions according to what I had found worthwhile to write down. However, such notes did not encapsulate her dimensionality (as shown by the productive directions *she* took us in by initiating sessions) despite her expectation that I would only find value in what she had "achieved" in our previous encounter. She was communicating this to me (and with me) through "process" before it was available to discuss as "content."

From one session to the next, there can be significant shifts in a patient's thoughts and feelings about the therapist. After all, we are only intermittently available to patients. We offer a conditional presence, predicated on a frame that *we* structure. It can be very painful to be in the midst of saying something meaningful and hear the provider say, "Time is up." Whatever is going on in the patient's mind needs to be dealt with alone until next time. The patient might feel angry, resentful, and even unwilling to "go through that again" when the next session comes. While we may be excited about the work done

---

[4] Bion was *not* suggesting we drop all memory of our patients from one session to the next, because this would be quite absurd and devaluing of the utility of the concept.

in one session and hope to go deeper next time, what happens after a particularly intense session might be anything *but* a seamless continuation. Patients might not show up, might arrive significantly late, or might rigidly keep sessions on a surface level, not going anywhere near the topics of last time. We can become discouraged when this happens, guiltily wondering if we did something wrong in the previous session to have caused the shift. What we have to offer, seemingly so useful before, suddenly feels less valuable.

A male therapist had a female patient who always started the sessions by discussing how his "psychobabble" was useless and how she had been trying to find alternatives to psychotherapy, such as self-help books and homeopathic remedies, which she felt contained all the answers she needed "without having to come here week after week and get nowhere." When it was queried what these alternatives could offer the patient, she fell silent, then muttered, "They don't kick me out." It was this dissatisfaction that had been finding its way into the beginnings of sessions, as the patient reintroduced her dropped and injured self to this therapist who had cut her off during their previous encounter. By listing her "alternative treatments," she made it known she could find a replacement therapist when needed (one more concretely under her control), viewing the "real" therapist as clumsy and inadequate, someone she did not need to miss after sessions ended. These strategies were ways of making separations and reapproximations more tolerable and less painful.

"Finding" the Transference

Talking about transference is both tantalizing and terrifying. It is touted as the epitome of "doing psychodynamic therapy." Yet we need to be careful about how we understand transference and what we do with this understanding.[5] We should not become obsessed with the transference or dismiss it. Just as we are always living out an object relationship with our patients, transference

---

[5] The sum of all the experiential components of how a patient relates to us is one way of thinking about the term *transference*. Melanie Klein used the term *total situation* to refer to the importance of keeping the transference in mind with all the patient's associations. She stated, "We are accustomed to speak of the transference situation. But do we always keep in mind the fundamental importance of this concept? It is my experience that in unravelling the details of the transference it is essential to think in terms of *total situations* transferred from the past into the present, as well as of emotions, defences and object-relations" (Klein 1952, p. 437, emphasis in original). A similarly broad view of countertransference can be applied. I have found Paula Heimann's definition to be the most succinct and useful: "I am using the term 'counter-transference' to cover all the feelings which the analyst experiences towards his patient" (Heimann 1950, p. 81).

and countertransference are always present. Thus, even in situations in which we are not openly discussing the transference, it is important to always try to keep it in mind. When appropriate, we seek ways to talk to the patient about what may be happening between the two of us.

Working in the displacement with patients can be immensely valuable, though one must be cognizant of its limitations. Working in the displacement typically involves processing with patients how they experience and interact with individuals in their everyday lives outside the therapy setting. During these conversations, patients might create detailed, play-by-play reconstructions of their interactions with other people, defending their own points of view, arguing how other persons were misguided or unfair, and sometimes even offering up "psychiatric diagnoses" they think are applicable to those they are describing. (Patients often ask if we agree with their take on matters.) Naturally, we are not directly privy to the relationships in question. We are only privy to the relationship patients have with *us*. As such, this is really the only one we can speak to, as much as there may be pressure on us to analyze all the other people in our patients' worlds.

It will likely become important to discuss transference dynamics at *some* point. Some may ask, "What is the point of discussing transference?" As Freud stated, "When all is said and done, it is impossible *to* destroy anyone *in absentia* or *in effigie*" (Freud 1912/1958, p. 108; emphasis in original). In other words, if there is a destructive relationship template dominating a patient's life, it will likely be futile to discuss concrete changes the patient can make in any outside relationships. Rather, it behooves us to try to notice and address how these damaging dynamics reemerge in the therapy sessions. The objective is not to concretely "fix" such ways of relating but rather to understand why they came to be *necessary*, as well as why they are being held onto and repeated. As much as we or our patients might try to make us out to be exceptions, we are *not* immune to the patient's internalized object world, and it will find its way into transference dynamics, in subtle or overt ways (or both).

When we are spoken about directly in sessions, it is important to allow space for patients to draw all sorts of conclusions about us, without feeling the need to "correct" them because the lens is too distorting. We might like to think we bring our empathic, funny, charming, and magnetic selves to the therapy room. However, patients will never get to know this "best self" of ours. It is hard enough for someone very close to us to appreciate us in the way we would like them to, let alone for this to happen in a relationship predicated on abstinence and neutrality. As much as we may be bringing a well-intentioned version of ourselves to sessions, patients may not view us that way at all. Rather, they will project onto us what *they* know from their internal object worlds, in interaction with elements they pick up from us and magnify according to assigned meaning (e.g., office setting, tone of voice, clothes, age, gender, race). What patients notice about us and how this resonates with their past experiences will inform who we become to them, for good or for ill (often, for both at the same time).

When we are working within a therapeutic model that favors transference explorations, psychoeducation about how such discussions can deepen the work is very important, at least at first. Although some might think that doing so may intellectualize and dilute the impact of transference-focused interventions, I am of the opinion that such education is in the service of transparency and fostering an alliance that can withstand the intensity of such exploration. Bringing up the relationship between therapist and patient in the course of a session, without an explanatory grounding having taken place at *any* point, can be distancing and alienating. Once the utility of transference explorations is outlined, the therapist is more freed up to engage in such conversations without needing to reiterate the reasoning for them. One could say, "Sometimes one way of understanding patterns that exist in outside relationships is to see in what ways they are also present here with us. If we notice something of these patterns being repeated in our interactions, we have the chance to talk about it in real time and think how we might work through it together." This will provide some grounding for patients; they might agree with this approach without knowing what it really entails, and our prefatory explanation may do little to mitigate the awkwardness of such conversations. Yet *somewhere* in their minds they will have a sense of where we are coming from when we make such incursions.

Sometimes trainees believe there is no transference. As I have stated, I do not believe this is ever the case. Whether the transference has become palpable or clear is a different matter, but we will always be *someone* to our patients, perceived and reacted to in accordance with their internal object worlds. If a patient has never directly shared personal feelings or thoughts about the therapist, it can feel awkward or anxiety-provoking for the latter to broach the topic. Indeed, when posed the question of how they feel about their therapist, patients might very well say, "I feel nothing about you." This in itself is grist for exploration—how can a patient share such intimate life details, week after week, yet have *no* thoughts or feelings about the person who has been listening this whole time? In thinking about a transference that looks barren, one can wonder with the patient where the feelings toward the therapist are to be found.

Similarly, sometimes transference interpretations can fall flat, making us feel like we were silly to have brought them up in the first place. However, this is where the "process versus content" matter is useful. An illustrative exchange follows.

T: I think what you are saying about your father applies to us. You say that
he never says anything that makes much sense to you, and you are left
feeling isolated and misunderstood. You may feel that's *me* when I say
things that show how little I understand about what's on your mind.

P: No, that's stupid. I'm talking about my father, not you.

T: There I go, saying something you feel makes no sense. I wonder what it's
like for you when I say stupid things.

Suddenly, it *is* about the transference. Although the initial comment might
have been hovering around the dominant theme and how it applied to our
dyad, it was not delivered on a level that would allow the patient to process
it. The object relationship needed to be *experienced* in the room, as opposed
to simply being thought about. In that moment, the therapist *became* the father, adopting his traits. The therapist's next intervention is an instance of
holding onto the projection and exploring, in the here and now, how these
interpersonal dynamics between the patient and "misunderstanding other"
are experienced.

Some therapists believe they have tried to address transference, only to
be summarily dismissed by a patient's lack of interest in the topic. Resigned
to the "impossibility" of having such a discussion, they might arrive at the
"solution" of cruising through subsequent sessions, never giving the matter
another thought. One male patient, enrolled in a resident clinic for several
years, seemed to be caught in a striking pattern that repeated itself with each
new resident who took over his care in July. Despite seeming to have a lot to
say and being capable of moments of remarkable introspection, this patient
invariably frustrated the residents, who thought he "teased" them with some
"good material" before closing himself back up. Several of them believed
"there is no transference coming from him" despite the paradoxically strong
*counter*transference response being evoked. Despite the gnawing feeling that
there was much richness beneath the surface, residents typically grew tired
of the dynamic and stopped investing energy in exploration. Subsequent
sessions would be dominated by surface and mind-numbing material until
the year ended and another resident could take over. The patient was never
kept for more than a year (though several residents had the chance to keep
him for another year). He was rarely chosen to be discussed in supervision,
being seen as a less "interesting" case. He had been raised in a family with
many siblings, with a father who worked three jobs and a mother who tried
desperately hard to provide for the children, both parents feeling constantly
spread thin. The patient never felt he actually had a place of his own in the
family unit, always thinking of himself as "number five of seven." He would
list other siblings as "the smart one," "the talented one," "the attractive one,"
"the funny one," and other appellations of uniqueness. His desire to locate the

aliveness inside himself and to find another person who would home in on what was special about *him* had been repeatedly frustrated. The parenting he received was mechanical and unemotional. Similarly, the pattern in therapy became one in which he was not a child worth knowing. Despite some initial investment, residents eventually became absentminded providers, just waiting until it was time to pass him along to the next "parent." Such a patient remained hidden in plain sight, desperate to be found (and perhaps desperate to remain hidden) but unable to produce the words needed to generate a response in the one listening. What had been thought of as a nonexistent transference was really one of devastating pathos.

Transference exploration takes trial and error, repetition, being made to feel stupid, making mistakes, finding ways in and being pushed away, and becoming hopeful with progress and then being dashed by resistance. It takes persistence. After all, we are attempting to find ways to *talk about* something that patients have only been able to live out. Critically, continued transference exploration may impact *outside* relationships, moving patients away from unthought repetition toward more thoughtful or creative forms of interacting, as patients take the insights gained from sessions into how they relate to others.

Is There a Process Behind Repetitive Content?

It is common for clinicians and patients to notice that certain topics are being constantly revisited during sessions, perhaps evoking the feeling that the narrative has not changed much over time. (Indeed, patients might make statements such as "I know I talk about this all the time" or "I feel like a broken record.") However, the fact that the same content keeps being repeated speaks to important aspects of the process. If a patient tells me, "I don't know why I keep bringing this up over and over again," I may respond with "Maybe because we haven't spoken about it *enough*" or "Maybe we need to figure out together what remains to be understood about it." In my language, I try to bring myself into the equation, moving from the "I" the patient used to the joint "we," implicating myself in the efforts to make sense of what the patient is saying, as well as in the failures to do so (which might be causing this content to recur). Creating a space in which particular content can be repeated without our becoming exasperated or discouraged can be very reassuring to patients and allow for small, gradual shifts over time. One patient with whom I had worked for several years told me that despite feeling he had failed to "crack open" certain areas of his life to gain "cognitive insight" into them, he *had* obtained a "visceral insight" into these areas, making them much more manageable. The improvements he noticed had taken place beyond conscious insights, suggesting that the very process of meeting has the potential to provide a level of containment. He had worried I would be like his adoptive parents, who showed disgust when he asked for their help with homework he could not understand. He would tell me, "If only they'd been patient with me, I think I'd have been able to come to a better understanding of how to do it. Instead, they dismissed me with such disdain.... I kept going back to the same problem over and over, with no greater knowledge of how to deal with it. If anything, I felt dumber." In our work, we needed to live through his worries of my becoming like the punitive object he had internalized. To do so, we survived hundreds of session-hours until there could be a reassurance provided on a visceral level, a process-driven containment transcending the domain of speech. For this containment to be felt, time and patience were necessary.

Clinical Vignettes

Vignette 1

In the vignette below, I outline the different directions a session might go in, depending on whether the therapist chooses to focus on content or process. Both approaches can be useful, but there will be a greater appreciation of the active object relationship in the room if the process is brought into awareness.

> P: After great deliberation, I didn't get you a gift for Christmas. I figured I don't know anything about you. I could've gotten you a box of tissues because of the ones I've used when I cry in here.
> T: The decision was made *not* to get me anything.
> P: It's like a "maybe next year" kind of thing because this will take forever.
> T: I wonder how you feel I'd react to receiving a gift from you.
> P: You're very quiet.... You'd probably just say, "Thank you," and that would be it....
> T: It wouldn't be spoken about any further.
> P: No.... I just remembered, I read something about this "deep stimulation."... I think it's "DBS" or something. Can't I just do that?
> T: Why?
> P: My brain...my brain, my brain. (She begins to speak rapidly about her upcoming trip to two exclusive spas in Italy and Austria in the company of several college friends.)

I will now present a hypothetical intervention that keeps the focus on the *content*. (Note that the extended, didactic phrasing of the therapist's statement does not represent how we would speak in an actual session; rather, it is used to illustrate more explicitly how content can guide clinical interventions. The same caveat applies to the later, process-focused intervention.)

T: You may feel as though you're condemned to be in treatment indefinitely, like your brother [diagnosed with "high-functioning autism spectrum disorder"], and only something dramatic from me—like DBS—can yield any results. You've commented on your brain being similar to his in the past. You speak about needing to escape; the only way to escape your fate is to be constantly on the move, going from one place to the next, along with people who don't have the brain issues that worry you so much.

P: I feel like I *am* him....I know I can't escape from myself, and I'm stuck with my own brain no matter what, even if I want to run away....It's just a fantasy, but I feel like I need to do it. I don't see how just talking about things can help, especially if I have a deeper issue beneath my "normal" appearance.

In contrast, a process-focused statement could be

T: There was a very quick transition from inside the room—the deliberation that went into getting me a gift or not, what I'd like, who I am, and how we will be invested in this process forever—to distant and dramatic departures—our treatment will be drastically interrupted by a trip, and even while you *are* here, it is better to do DBS and magically transform your brain rather than do therapy. Perhaps in anticipation of our separation next month, there's a need to create distance.

P: There's a lot on my mind....I feel guilty about not getting you a gift. I also sometimes *don't* get people gifts as a way of showing them I hate them. I could bake you a pie, but I wouldn't blame you for throwing it away....I could be poisoning you, you know....

As one can appreciate, the relationship becomes *much* more alive with the second intervention because it draws the therapist in closer as a real object in the room.

Vignette 2 (The "Process" of Telling a Dream)

Dream interpretation has been hailed as the "royal road to a knowledge of the unconscious" (Freud 1900/1953, p. 608). When the significance of dreams is being explored, the focus is almost invariably on their symbolic, "content" value. However, there is a "process" to how and when dreams are reported in sessions that extends their clinical relevance beyond their overt content (Ermann 1999). A patient started a 3:00 P.M. session by saying, "I need to end at 3:58, as I have a meeting at 4." A bit surprised by the patient's words, given the well-established parameter of ending at 50 minutes, the therapist stated, "Oh, we'll end around 3:50 P.M." The patient's use of the pronoun *I* and of the verb *need* perhaps carried more weight than could be initially appreciated. The patient was expressing perhaps an unconscious need for the therapist to bend the frame, to be an object that could be accessed beyond the restrictions imposed by reality. When the therapist, at 3:50, stated, "We're out of time," the patient responded by offering up a very provocative dream (which was recounted rather quickly): "Oh wait, I forgot to tell you—I had a dream last night that I was being bludgeoned to death by an authority figure sitting in a judge's chair....What does it mean?" One could go in a number of directions with this. One could be drawn in by the content; after all, the patient had given the therapist the "gift" of 8 more minutes during which such a compelling dream could be discussed. The provider would thus become the "3:58 therapist," living up to the role of an all-good object, one that allows the patient to determine what measure of reality is tolerable, including when sessions end. Also, the therapist would hardly want to align with that dreaded, all-bad object from the dream, the authority figure who was attacking the patient with those judgmental "rules."

Despite these pressures, the therapist observed the frame, saying, "That's very important. We'll talk about it next week if you like." The session ended. The presentation of the dream, with all its intriguing content, was likely an attempt to undo the imposing frame of the therapist, underlining the need to keep the process in mind when listening to dream material.

KEY POINTS

- The "content" of a session corresponds to the spoken words said by patient and therapist. The "process" of a session denotes the action language—the implicit, largely nonverbal dynamic that unfolds during the encounter.

- How patients carry themselves in sessions can help us understand how we are being viewed at any given moment. This invites the very useful question "What type of object am I to this patient at this time?"

- If we are viewed as an inviting, interested object, we may notice this in a patient's relaxed body language and mode of speaking. Alternatively, if we are viewed as harsh or judgmental, we may notice a tense, "shutting-down" communicative style. Critically, these considerations will be reflected in, yet also transcend, the content dimension of communication.

- The process of being with a patient can often help us viscerally sense the pressure to behave as or identify with an internal object, one based on a figure from a patient's early life.

References

Bergstein A: Violent emotions and the violence of life. Int J Psychoanal 101(5):863–878, 2020 33952134

Bion W: Attention and Interpretation (1970). Oxford, UK, Rowman & Littlefield, 2004

Chefetz R: Dignity is the opposite of shame, and pride is the opposite of guilt. Attachment: New Directions in Psychotherapy and Relational Psychoanalysis 11:119–133, 2017

Ermann M: Telling dreams and transference. International Forum of Psychoanalysis 8:75–86, 1999

Freud S: The interpretation of dreams (first part) (1900), in The Standard Edition of the Complete Psychological Works of Sigmund Freud, Vol 4. Translated and edited by Strachey J. London, Hogarth Press, 1953, pp ix–627

Freud S: Fragment of an analysis of a case of hysteria (1905 [1901]), in The Standard Edition of the Complete Psychological Works of Sigmund Freud, Vol 7. Translated and edited by Strachey J. London, Hogarth Press, 1953, pp 1–122

Freud S: The dynamics of transference (1912), in The Standard Edition of the Complete Psychological Works of Sigmund Freud, Vol 12. Translated and edited by Strachey J. London, Hogarth Press, 1958, pp 97–108

Freud S: On beginning the treatment (further recommendations on the technique of psycho-analysis I) (1913), in The Standard Edition of the Complete Psychological Works of Sigmund Freud, Vol 12. Translated and edited by Strachey J. London, Hogarth Press, 1958, pp 121–144

Freud S: Negation (1925), in The Standard Edition of the Complete Psychological Works of Sigmund Freud, Vol 19. Translated and edited by Strachey J. London, Hogarth Press, 1961, pp 233–240

Heimann P: On counter-transference. Int J Psychoanal 31:81–84, 1950

Isaacs S: The nature and function of phantasy. Int J Psychoanal 29:73–97, 1948

Klein M: The origins of transference. Int J Psychoanal 33(4):433–438, 1952 12999365

Stern DN, Sander LW, Nahum JP, et al: Non-interpretive mechanisms in psychoanalytic therapy: the "something more" than interpretation. Int J Psychoanal 79 (Pt 5):903–921, 1998 9871830

Developing a Sense of Self: Theory

When I was One,
I had just begun.

When I was Two,
I was nearly new.

When I was Three,
I was hardly me.

A.A. Milne, "The End" (Milne 1927/1988)

I've always thought that children are much wiser than us (…) For me, children somehow connect our world with another world, a transcendent world to which they haven't yet lost their connection. They will soon, but they haven't yet. (…) When a grown-up can't find words to express something, I think he should ask a child. The child will be able to clarify everything, even just by his presence.

Andrei Tarkovsky (2019)

IN THIS AND the following four chapters, I will present more advanced concepts pertaining to object relations theory and practice, drawing extensively from the psychodynamic literature and from other scientific realms to outline the factors in early life that shape how one views the self and relates to others. As argued in this book, the objects in one's environment will play a crucial role in such developments.

Different theorists have unique approaches to outlining the conflicts and milestones believed to be inherent to distinct age periods over the life cycle. One of the better-known examples is Freud's psychosexual staging of development, starting with the first 18 months of life (oral stage) and progressing through early adolescence (genital stage) (Freud 1905/1953). Erik Erikson delineated the various "negotiations" taking place during discrete age ranges, starting with "trust versus mistrust" (in the first year of life) and culminating with the final stage of "integrity versus despair" in sexagenarians, ostensibly lasting until the end of their lives (Erikson 1959/1980).[1] There is a wonderful body of literature on the different stages of life and their psychodynamic underpinnings; indeed, such descriptions have informed much of how we conceptualize the demands, obstacles, joys, disappointments, and conflicts that emerge as time goes by. Interested readers are encouraged to delve into the literature on latency, adolescence, adulthood, and aging (Blos 1967; Greenberg 2009; Novick and Novick 1994; Quinodoz 2010).

As opposed to adopting a linear, stage-wise approach to development, I will be aligning my thoughts with the Kleinian and object relations perspective. The first five chapters in this book presented a more "gestalt" approach to object relations theory, with the intention of outlining some basic concepts to allow initial immersion into the work of outpatient psychotherapy. In this and the next three chapters, I delve into the developmental factors informing how a sense of self and object relatedness evolve during early life.

Timelines of Dyadic and Triadic Relating

Child-caregiver dyadic interactions are critical in early life, shaping the child's development of a sense of self and others. Through part-object relating (see Chapter 1, "Introduction")—characteristic of the earlier, paranoid-schizoid position—a child discovers split-off and projected parts of the self in the attuned caregiver, who welcomes the child's projections. A concerned caregiver gives the child the containing presence that is needed to make sense of a world of sensory bombardment, both from within and from without. As the child *feels* this containment, scaffolded by the nurturance of benign, loving external objects, discomfort and frustration can be better tolerated. In tandem with the child's developing motor and cognitive skills, the ability to view the world in more nuanced and complex ways also emerges, as projections lessen and the child is better able to hold onto different as-

---

[1] In addition to the eight stages outlined by Erikson, his wife Joan Erikson later proposed a ninth stage, reflecting on how several previously negotiated conflicts would be revisited when people were in their 80s and 90s.

pects of the self without trying to be rid of them. As this unfolds, the child moves from a predominantly dyadic (part-object) configuration to a *triadic* one (made up of whole objects). In this progression, there is an evolving awareness that the external object has relationships with other objects, *excluding* the child. Learning to negotiate triangulation is the major task of the Oedipal situation, which I align with depressive position dynamics and place after age 3 years; this occurs along with the child's ability to internalize the *function* of the containing object (gradually lessening the need for physical presence) and neurobiologically activate areas involved in mentalization, allowing for nuanced, alternative perspectives to be considered, beyond the simplicity of splitting.

I am aware that a number of academics and clinicians may take issue with my grouping pre-Oedipal dynamics with Klein's paranoid-schizoid position and Oedipal dynamics with her depressive position. After all, there is *not* a perfect temporal overlap between Klein's characterization of the paranoid-schizoid position (which she dated as occurring during the first 4–6 months of age) and Freud's oral (0–18 months) and anal (18–36 months) stages. However, my alignment has didactic, neuroscientific, and clinical merit. It also carries a level of intuitive logic when we consider how a person's development sequentially advances from two-person to three-person, a progression that seems quite apropos for how typical immersion into the societal fabric takes place. We may move from interacting with a parent or caregiver to both parents or caregivers, the larger family unit, other family units, and society at large, in stepwise manners. In doing so, we discover how we as individuals are perceived and positioned by those with whom we interact.

The two-person mode of relating is narrow in its scope, with a predominance of splitting and projective mechanisms. In projecting parts of the self into an object and observing how the latter is impacted, the projector is able to gain a more immediate and cause-and-effect sense of the nature of one's projected traits and the influence they have on those around. In the early environment of the developing child, such interactions (and their outcomes) are critical for determining how the world will be patterned and internalized in terms of working models of self and others. There is a level of sensed control over the object in dyadic interactions because one is relating largely through the use of projected parts of self, in a way keeping the "otherness" of the object's mind largely unseen. Under the sway of strong projections, the illusion is sustained that the object can be completely controlled (omnipotence) and known (omniscience). Such an illusion is not pathological but rather an important and necessary initial step in a child's development because too much unpredictability in an undeveloped mind could lead to impossible confusion and failure to integrate the meaning of early life experiences.

The three-person mode of relating is endlessly complicated; it acknowledges the passing of time and the essential mutability of object relationships. In this mode, omnipotence and omniscience are impossibilities because knowledge is never complete, and our minds need to be constantly open to assimilating new information. After all, when I say "three-person," the "third" is essentially that which is beyond one's control: objects now have minds of their own, ones that cannot be reduced to the workings of projections. Hence, the reassurance provided by dyadic forms of relating is no longer present. Negotiating this triangular space is a lifelong endeavor and one that acquires renewed salience as one is confronted with the inevitability of accumulating losses and the need to acknowledge one's limitations in life. Although we may cultivate the notion that we are exceptions to nature's designs of aging and losing specialness, this is gradually shed away in the depressive position. This entails mourning the idealized version of the world and of oneself and accepting that others have relationships that may be equally or more enticing than the ones they have with us. This can be profoundly painful yet also quite liberating and growth-promoting when seen for its potential benefits.

As I mentioned earlier, I am not presenting a stepwise approach to development that encompasses the life cycle in a linear progression through age-defined conflicts. Rather, what I wish to emphasize is this: one does not "progress" through the paranoid-schizoid position and never go back. There is a fluctuation between paranoid-schizoid and depressive position dynamics over the course of one's life. Fundamentally, it is the shift between these two positions that grounds object relations theory. This might seem like a simplification of psychic functioning, but there is an immense complexity contained in both of these positions, as I hope to illustrate. Most important, maintaining this frame in mind will allow for us to understand what the working object relationship in the room is at a given time (i.e., how a patient is viewing self and therapist) and how we may be able to link these active dynamics with developmental factors from the patient's early life.

I will now present a theoretical understanding of the development of self, beginning somewhat more broadly and then narrowing my descriptions primarily to the theories of Winnicott, Klein, and Bion. I do this to highlight the useful correlations between advances in our scientific understanding of child development and the keen insights posited by psychoanalytic practitioners years before.

Development of Self

The task of early development is to establish a sense of who one is in the world. In the young child, it is through preverbal and somatically informed experiences that a working map of one's environment is established. Early experiences of containment rely on sensory awareness and receptivity by the caregiver, the use of language being a later, more advanced dimension of interpersonal communication. The very word *infant* derives from the Latin *infantem* (nominative *infans*), a noun use of an adjective meaning "not able to speak."

If adequate and attuned caregiving takes place, a basic sense of safety emerges, empowering the child to "run with" evolving psychomotor abilities in playful, exploratory ways. The converse occurs when such attunement does *not* take place and, despite physical body growth, there is inhibition in emotional and cognitive development, given the lack of sensed safety in the environment. What should be explicitly stated here is that *the development of self is inextricably linked with the nature and quality of one's interactions with early objects*. This view aligns with the argument that genetic endowment is not fatalistic in determining particular outcomes; rather, it is a substrate *on which* the environment will act, leading to different gene expression patterns and phenotypes depending on what type of world the individual encounters (Belsky 1997; Belsky et al. 2007, 2009). As such, who one is cannot be separated from who one is in relation to the world; how early objects view and interact with a child become part of this child's internalized view of self. This informs Winnicott's celebrated statement "There is no such thing as an infant" (Winnicott 1960, p. 587), indicating that a baby never exists in isolation but in relation to one's surroundings. Even if there is no one around, this is still (and perhaps, even *more* of) a critical consideration in influencing development. Babies who grow up with severe deprivation and limited contact may display profound emotional and cognitive delays; this was evidenced in a series of studies of children raised in adoptive homes after suffering terrible deprivation in Romanian orphanages and showing enduring effects on their neuropsychiatric health (Chugani et al. 2001; Eluvathingal et al. 2006; Kumsta et al. 2010, 2015; Mackes et al. 2020). Indeed, in severe cases, children displayed a "quasi-autistic" syndrome (Rutter et al. 2007). Having a caregiver who is attuned and responsive is not merely a consideration for laying down a sense of environmental safety versus risk. Rather, it is a *critical* dimension determining brain, motor, and neuroendocrine development; lack of such environmental factors may severely impair the child in ways that may not be entirely reversible, even with adequate subsequent rearing.

When there *is* proper involvement, children will necessarily be turning to their caregivers to make sense of a world that is impossibly vast and overwhelming. Assimilating information about one's environment is done piecemeal, in tandem with the child's limitations and abilities to grasp what is being encountered. Nature is very wise in this sense, and indeed what needs to be negotiated moves from fundamentally dyadic considerations to increasingly broader levels of engagement. For instance, an infant's visual acuity at birth can be as low as 20/800, probably enough to see the nipple right in front of one's eyes but not much more (Shapiro et al. 2017, p. 3362).

Using the caregiver as a sounding board will be a critical process in trying to take in the sensory bombardment with which the child is faced. What has been termed *social referencing* is an example. This can be somewhat narrowly defined as looking to adults for emotional and behavioral cues when faced with ambiguous situations, seeking guidance as to how one should resolve the scenario. After all, when uncertainty arises, the child looks to a trusted figure, one wiser and stronger than the self. Social referencing can lead to a child patterning which responses are "most appropriate" when something similar arises in the future. This essentially grafts an adult's form of handling an event onto the child's own thought process, with the child immediately identifying with the adult's way of operating. Self and other become indistinguishable in such instances.

As an evocative example of this dynamic, the "visual cliff" was devised by psychologists Eleanor Gibson and Richard Walk. It consisted of a Plexiglas sheet that covered a checkerboard-pattern cloth. The latter was placed under the Plexiglas up to a certain point, giving the impression of "solid ground" underneath; then the cloth would suddenly appear to have "dropped" 4 feet down. The Plexiglas would be intact, but the discontinuity in the cloth pattern gave the impression of a precipitous drop. One study assessed how 1-year-olds negotiated this visual cliff (Sorce et al. 1985). Children were placed at one end of the table, where the Plexiglas and cloth gave the impression of a firm floor underneath. The child's mother was positioned at the other end of the table. The child would begin to crawl toward the mother, up until the area of the Plexiglas where the cloth patterning appeared to have dropped; here, children might worry about falling if they were to continue moving forward, despite feeling the sturdiness of the Plexiglas. At this threshold, the child looks to the mother. If the latter gives encouraging signs to continue, the child will do so, crossing the cliff over to her. If, however, the mother looks frightened or concerned, the child will remain at the threshold and not cross the cliff, having received the message that it is dangerous to do so.

Behaviorally modeling oneself on others can also lead to overtly destructive outcomes. In the 1960s, Canadian psychologist Albert Bandura conducted a series of experiments involving children ages 37–69 months (Bandura 1965; Bandura et al. 1963). In his studies, children observed adults hitting a Bobo doll (a toy with a rounded bottom and a low center of mass, allowing it to rock back to an upright position after being knocked down).

In the experiments, adults could be rewarded or punished for these behaviors. In a model supporting observational learning, Bandura noted that children would mimic the aggressive behaviors of the adults, especially if the latter did not incur punishment for their actions. (Of note, this imitation occurred whether the child witnessed the adult attacking the doll in person or on film, raising the polemical question of whether violence in the media influences real-life aggressive tendencies.)[2]

These findings underline the significance of nonverbal and behavioral dimensions to providing a child with a sense of how the surrounding environment operates, as well as with implicit guidance as to how to behave, which can become ineluctably identified with one's ingrained sense of self. This can prove problematic, especially when identification with an abusive or erratic caregiver is adopted as a solution to a chaotic surround.

I will now discuss the "facilitative" and "interactive" dimensions influencing a child's development of self, while bringing in relevant theory from psychoanalytic models. This breakdown is my own and is used to aid readers with assimilating these theoretical viewpoints. Although there are more nuances and greater overlap than will be presented here, didactic and practical clarity are the main considerations, though conceptual integrity has not been compromised in the process.

Facilitative Dimensions

When I speak of "facilitative" dimensions, I am referring to an environment that essentially provides a supportive surround, allowing children to develop as closely as possible to their full potential. An attuned caregiver welcomes and meets the spontaneous gesture of the child, allowing the latter to be expressive without undue limitation or impingement by the object. Winnicott wrote extensively on how an optimal environment provides sufficient scaffolding for a child to develop without experiencing premature constrictions. Winnicott used the term *holding* to characterize the physical and emotional care provided by an infant's parent (the mother, in his descriptions) (Winnicott 1953, 1956/1992, 1960). In effect, the parent's sensitive caregiving facilitates gradual consolidation of the infant's psychosomatic sense of being, which is experienced in unintegrated and incomplete manners during early life. Such caregiving meets the child's physiological needs and provides pro-

---

[2] The findings by Bandura were in children older than those in the age range I am focusing on in this chapter, but they are included to illustrate how "taking in" what we observe from others can guide our own moral compass throughout life. (Bandura's model served as a basis for what was later termed *moral disengagement*.)

tection from overwhelming stimuli, actively adapting to the child's requirements. In such conditions, whatever frustrations *do* take place are limited
and kept within the bounds of what is tolerable to the child. Through such
sensitive holding, children begin to develop an awareness of their own bodies in relation to the outside world and to others, slowly making sense of
unintegrated bits of experience. An experience of continuity in a child is dependent on three interacting factors: 1) sense of safety in the inner world
(given the presence of an internal good object), 2) an ability to limit concern
with external events, and 3) the generation of spontaneous creative gestures
(Winnicott 1958/1965). Regarding the third point, the parent needs to be
open and receptive to a child's spontaneity, creativity, and playfulness, man-
ifestations of the child's individuality and "true self." A parent's flexible and
soft response allows for a sense of dyadic attunement to emerge, giving
scope and meaning to the child's expressions. These instances, which are
highly structuring for the child, arise from what Winnicott termed "primary
maternal preoccupation" (Winnicott 1956/1992), wherein the mother offers
the baby the "illusion" that she is an extension of the baby, an external object
created by the latter (this can be thought of as a form of "magical omnipotence").[3] Winnicott believed this was a *necessary* stepping stone in healthy development: "The mother's eventual task is gradually to disillusion the
infant, but she has no hope of success unless at first she has been able to give
sufficient opportunity for illusion" (Winnicott 1953, p. 95).

Importantly, in this same paper, Winnicott developed the concept of
transitional phenomena (which we have come to term *transitional objects*). In its
common acceptation, a child may carry around an item such as a teddy bear
or a blanket because of its felt associations with the soothing function provided by a caregiver, who is not always physically around to attend to the child.
The transitional object serves to concretely help the child move from requiring a more contingent caregiver presence to being able to internalize and exercise more autonomously the soothing *function* of the caregiver.

However, transitional objects serve an earlier, more primitive function
for the young child, helping to distinguish between "me" and "not-me" because these objects will be imbued with projections from the child (thus being seen as part of the self) while also being objectively perceived as "other."
Dealing with transitional objects also affords some level of omnipotence to
the child, who can throw away and retrieve the object at will, gaining a sense
of the bounds of oneself in more controlled ways than those allowed by real

---

[3] Although Winnicott ascribed these functions to the mother, we can apply the concept to fathers, extended family, and alloparents, depending on who is in a primary
caregiver role for an infant.

objects with minds of their own.[4] Winnicott (1953) stated, "The transitional object and the transitional phenomena start each human being off with what will always be important for them, i.e., a neutral area of experience which will not be challenged" (p. 95).

As me/not-me boundaries are increasingly consolidated (through live and transitional objects), the child progresses from "object-relating" to "object-usage" (Winnicott 1969). This is a move from relating to objects as "a bundle of projections" (p. 712) to using or viewing the object in a fuller, whole manner. (This is akin to the transition from part-object to whole-object relationships.)

Of course, no caregiver can be fully attuned or receptive all the time. Nor is this desirable, because some aliquot of frustration is *necessary* to foster healthy development. In learning to negotiate the inevitable separateness of important objects, the child is implicitly granted "permission" to also exist as a separate person, beyond dyadic constraints. Thus, for Winnicott, the operant concept is not that of a perfect parent but rather of a "good-enough" parent. He states, "The good-enough mother meets the omnipotence of the infant and to some extent makes sense of it. She does this repeatedly. A True Self begins to have life, through the strength given to the infant's weak ego by the mother's implementation of the infant's omnipotent expressions" (Winnicott 1960/1965, p. 145).

Importantly, it is through "optimal" frustrations that children discover their own potential and limitations. A child is better able to tolerate giving up feelings of omnipotence when this is done gradually. Child development research indicates that moderate degrees of maternal involvement are *preferable* to highly contingent responses, with healthier relating patterns being observed at follow-up (Forcada-Guex et al. 2006; Malatesta et al. 1989). When provided with an *optimally facilitating environment* by such sensitive caregiving, children are better able to understand their own unique and individual abilities, consolidating a more realistic sense of self. This is akin to

---

[4] We are reminded of Freud's description of the game played by a 1.5-year-old child, in which a wooden reel would be tossed away (accompanied by the child saying the German word *fort* ["gone"]) and then pulled back by an attached string (the child then joyfully saying *da* ["there"]). Freud hypothesized that the child developed this game as a way of mastering instances of separation from his mother. He stated, "This, then, was the complete game—disappearance and return (…) though there is no doubt that the greater pleasure was attached to the second act. The interpretation of the game then became obvious. It was related to the child's great cultural achievement—the instinctual renunciation (that is, the renunciation of instinctual satisfaction) which he had made in allowing his mother to go away without protesting. He compensated himself for this, as it were, by himself staging the disappearance and return of the objects within his reach" (Freud 1920/1955, p. 15).

the "zone of proximal development" described by psychologist Lev Vygotsky (Vygotsky 1978), defined as the difference between what a learner can do without help from the environment and what can be done when help is offered (Figure 6–1). Although this was described for schoolchildren and is arguably a variation of "meeting the learners where they are at" (i.e., presenting knowledge in assimilable ways based on the child's developmental level), we see parallels between what he proposed and the facilitative aspects of caregiving that allow a child's full potential to be cultivated.

There is more to the caregiver's function than providing an environment in which a child's expressiveness is facilitated. During moments of distress, the attuned caregiver helps process the unbearable state the child may be in. As Winnicott stated,

> I do not believe it is possible to understand the functioning of the mother at the very beginning of the infant's life without seeing that she must be able to reach this state of heightened sensitivity, almost an illness, and to recover from it. (...) Only if a mother is sensitized in the way I am describing can she feel herself into her infant's place, and so meet the infant's needs. (Winnicott 1956/1992, pp. 302, 304)

Establishing an environment that protects the child from excessive stimuli has been likened to a "shield" limiting what is experienced by the child's immature sensorium. Freud discussed the concept of a protective shield (*Reizschutz*) that serves as a barrier to fend off excessive stimulation to a living organism. He stated, "*Protection against* stimuli is an almost more important function for the living organism than *reception of* stimuli" (Freud 1920/1955, p. 27; emphasis in original). He went on to describe as *traumatic* "any excitations from outside which are powerful enough to break through the protective shield" (p. 29). Masud Khan, a Pakistani-British psychoanalyst who elaborated on Winnicott's theories, likened the role of the mother to that of this protective shield, keeping the child from being exposed to damaging stimuli. (I argue that this applies to any primary caregiver [given the many different figures who may be involved in rearing], not exclusively to the maternal role.) Khan elaborates:

> [C]umulative trauma is the result of the breaches in the mother's role as a protective shield over the whole course of the child's development, from infancy to adolescence—that is to say, in all those areas of experience where the child continues to need the mother as an auxiliary ego to support his immature and unstable ego functions. (Khan 1963, p. 290)

Freud recognized that what a child might be responding to as external stimuli may be deriving from a projection of one's own *internal* state. The pro-

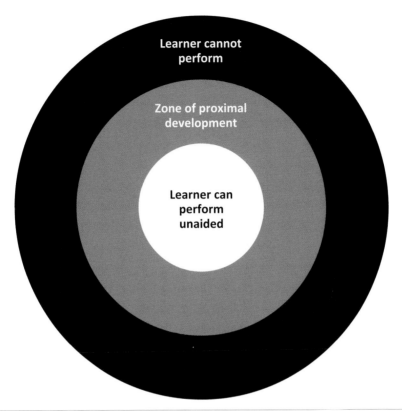

Figure 6–1.   Schematic depiction of Vygotsky's zone of proximal
development.

tective shield is less effective against internal stimuli; one way of handling unpleasant inner excitations is to project them outward, "as though they were acting, not from the inside, but from the outside, so that it may be possible to bring the shield against stimuli into operation as a means of defense against them. This is the origin of *projection*, which is destined to play such a large part in the causation of pathological processes" (Freud 1920/1955, p. 29; emphasis in original). We can thereby see how external objects can become "bad objects," experienced as the causers of distress. When the caregiver is able to attune to the child's internal state, these projections are metabolized and can be reintegrated by the child not as something potentially life-threatening but rather as an experience that can be managed and survived, as modeled by the external object.

Unfortunately, a *lack* of containing experiences may be the norm in a child's early life. If the caregiver is *not* responsive to the child's gestures, protection from excessive stimuli is not provided, and the child is left feeling overwhelmed and without any recourse left to deal with discomfort, pathological solutions may emerge. I have already discussed the genesis of splitting and how its rigidity can significantly narrow the scope of object relating. In Winnicott's view, when the object shows a lack of interest or concern in a child's expressions (as opposed to openly welcoming them), the result may be that the child will learn to shut down any "true self" gestures and behave in more superficial, two-dimensional ways. Given the need to preserve the attachment with the provider, even at the expense of one's own emotional expression, the child may become highly attentive to what the caregiver finds tolerable, mimicking attributes or adopting behaviors that seem to keep things calmer and more predictable. In the process, important dimensions of the child's selfhood may be sacrificed, given the unfavorable conditions for playful self-discovery. There is little room for complex emotional expression and a pacing of psychic growth. Rather, the child needs to adapt quickly to the demands of the environment, identifying with the needs and wants of adult figures without the cognitive tools to make sense of them, resulting in a form of "pseudomaturity." The child's mind and behaviors do not evolve; rather, sameness is painfully maintained at the expense of subjective and individual richness. This precocious adaptation is the essence of the "false self." As Winnicott stated,

> The mother who is not good enough is not able to implement the infant's omnipotence, and so she repeatedly fails to meet the infant gesture; instead she substitutes her own gesture which is to be given sense by the compliance of the infant. This compliance on the part of the infant is the earliest stage of the False Self, and belongs to the mother's inability to sense her infant's needs. (Winnicott 1960/1965, p. 145)

While Winnicott stated that *some* degree of "false self" expression is necessary to function in civilized society, if it is overly organizing, there will be little room for the "true self" to be accessed and expressed. This may lead to a sense of alienation from oneself and to a feeling of phoniness when relating to others. Winnicott said the "false self" has a "very important function: to hide the True Self, which it does by compliance with environmental demands" (Winnicott 1960/1965, pp. 146–147).

It has been argued, perhaps unfairly, that Winnicott's thinking may be too optimistic because one might infer that as long as the environment is ideal, the child's best self will inevitably be expressed. Although Winnicott did *not* deny the aggressive aspects of the infant, he did seem to view them as a more mysterious human disposition than love and affiliation. Even when he *does* speak of hatred and destructiveness, he often couches them in more hopeful terms. He recognized that love and hate "form the two chief elements out of which human affairs are built" (Winnicott 1939/1964, p. 73). However, an infant's hatred and capacity for destruction are presented as 1) something that will trigger a protective urge toward the loved object, "and the main destruction must always exist in his fantasy" (p. 76); 2) deriving originally from an excitation, an urge to move or expend energy, or an unsatisfied appetite; and 3) something that can become manifest when there is not a safer alternative form of "disposing of badness" (p. 78).[5] As the second and third points suggest, there is a failure in the environment to present appropriate options for the child to express the self in healthy ways, as well as a failure to satisfy the child's immediate needs or appetites. Through this lens, even *primary* aggression would be "in reaction to" or "secondary to" the child's unsatisfying experience of the surround.

I will expand somewhat more on the idea of a child's aggressiveness in the next section, focusing on the work of Klein, who had a considerably different perspective on children's constitutional hatred and capacity for destruction.

Interactive Dimensions

KLEIN AND THE PARANOID-SCHIZOID POSITION

In Chapter 1, I outlined the defense mechanisms attendant on early life (i.e., splitting and projective identification) while also differentiating between part-object and whole-object relating. In this section (and in Chapter 8, "The Oedipal Situation [Exclusion and Rivalry]: Theory"), I will integrate these concepts within the framework of Klein's two positions: paranoid-schizoid (PS) and depressive (D).

In the paranoid-schizoid position, one is in a state of relative unintegration, splitting off and projecting into objects bits of one's inner world, maintaining a dyadic link wherein a clear sense of boundaries is effaced, as others may be experienced as concretely holding parts of the self. In the later, depressive position, integration is greater. One is able to appreciate self and others in fuller ways (without resorting to excessive projection), entertain nuance and contradiction, and allow objects to exist as separate entities (without this being threatening to one's sense of self).

To reiterate, there is a back-and-forth between these two positions throughout life. We are constantly oscillating between mind-states in which we are able to entertain complexity and uncertainty and ones in which doubt and alternative perspectives are jettisoned in favor of absolute ways of think-

---

[5] Readers are referred to Winnicott's paper "The Use of an Object" (Winnicott 1969) for a thought-provoking exploration of a child's inherent destructiveness.

ing. When faced with distressing circumstances, we might notice ourselves becoming "undone" for a bit before transitioning back to a more depressive mode. Someone left by a romantic partner, for instance, may experience a pull toward a state of psychic disintegration, being invaded by despair and the feeling that life is now empty and bereft of meaning. When faced with the loss of a significant other, one might project one's entire sense of worth into the (now former) partner, impoverishing the self, even if up until that point the relationship seemed to be healthy and mature, with each person maintaining a sense of individuality that was not sacrificed for the sake of the attachment. Grief can impel the individual toward paranoid-schizoid dynamics; indeed, this may be what *needs* to take place, at least for a bit, as the loss is deeply felt and processed. The hope is that the individual will be able to move back toward a state of integration and independent functioning, reclaiming a sense of worth that is not limited to the confines of one's past relationships and reestablishing one's own value as a whole object. This is one example of how these dynamics are relevant to adult life.

The task in childhood is to experience moments of relative disintegration and recover from them with the aid of an attuned object who joins with the child in the latter's psychic reality and helps make it tolerable. Over time, repeated experiences of dyadic integration provide the basis for the working-through of the depressive position, wherein the child is able to use the "function" learned from the parent or caregiver and self-soothe when threatened with stress or frustration. As elaborated by Bion, the back and forth between the two positions is an organizing principle of psychic life, depicted as PS $\leftrightarrow$ D (Bion 1963/2018).[6] Recognizing the dynamic quality of these modes of mental functioning, Klein opted for the term *position* as opposed to *phase*. One does not "graduate" from either position and never face it again.

Klein elaborated on these two positions over the course of her career. In "A Contribution to the Psychogenesis of Manic Depressive States" (Klein 1935/ 1975), she discussed the concept of "positions" ("paranoiac" [the original term for paranoid-schizoid] and depressive), as well as part- and whole-objects. In subsequent works, these concepts became better consolidated. In "Notes on Some Schizoid Mechanisms," she discussed in greater detail the paranoid-schizoid position and the anxieties or defensive structures pertaining to this mode of functioning (Klein 1946).

As mentioned, the paranoid-schizoid position is characterized by predominantly part-object relating—dyadic configurations in which the child is constantly projecting into and introjecting from the object, such that where self ends and other begins is not clearly delineated. This is immersion in a

---

[6] See Chapter 8.

sensory world predating cognitive, symbolic understanding. If a terrible sensation is felt in the body, the child might feel as though the self is being destroyed by some oppressive force, which may be perceived as coming from the outside through projection. When the mother is the recipient, she will become a persecuting figure (the bad object described previously), suffused as she is with the child's projected aggression (Klein 1933/1975, 1958; Segal 1988). As such, the young child is, from the outset, threatened with annihilation both from within and without. This anti-life, experiential sense of annihilating destructiveness has been termed the "death drive" or "death instinct."[7] As Klein stated,

> I hold that anxiety arises from the operation of the Death Instinct within the organism, is felt as fear of annihilation (death) and takes the form of fear of persecution. The fear of the destructive impulse seems to attach itself at once to an object—or rather it is experienced as fear of an uncontrollable overpowering object. Other important sources of primary anxiety are the trauma of birth (separation anxiety) and frustration of bodily needs; and these experiences too are from the beginning felt to be caused by bad objects. Even if these objects are felt to be external, they become through introjection internal persecutors and thus reinforce the fear of the destructive impulse within. (Klein 1946, p. 100)

The counterpart to these terrifying forces is the idealized, all-giving, all-good object, which is desperately needed to provide *some* semblance of integration. Experiencing an external object as all good is similarly predicated on the child's projecting something of the self into it; thus, the "good" is felt to be coming from an outside source. As mentioned, predominance of "good" over "bad" experiences gradually allows the child to take back projected aspects, imbuing oneself with a greater sense of wholeness and acquiring a more nuanced and realistic appreciation of the qualities of external objects, none of which are *only* good or bad. So, what might interfere with this taking place?

---

[7] Most theorists reject the notion of a primary death instinct; Klein was one of the few to expand on it. Freud initially described it in 1920 (in "Beyond the Pleasure Principle") and returned to the idea in later works. It is a concept that has generated confusion and controversy, some equating it with the tendency humans have toward self-destructive and suicidal behaviors. However, Freud's conceptualization was less clear-cut in its implications; he aligned the death drive with a return to a prior state of being, one of inertia and minimal excitation. Borrowing from an (arguably incorrect) interpretation of Buddhist thought, he used the term "Nirvana Principle" to characterize this "effort to reduce, to keep constant or to remove internal tension due to stimuli" (Freud 1920/1955, pp. 55–56). In reaching ultimate quiescence, life itself would essentially be eradicated.

ENVY

> *Hate, as a relation to objects, is older than love.(…) [I]t always re-*
> *mains in an intimate relation with the self-preservative instincts.*
>
> Sigmund Freud (1915/1957, p. 139)

> *It is certain that envy is the worst sin that is; for all other sins are*
> *sins only against one virtue, whereas envy is against all virtue and*
> *against all goodness.*
>
> Klein (1957/1975, p. 189) (quoting from Chaucer's
> *The Canterbury Tales*)[8]

One of the most controversial topics in psychoanalytic theory is the concept of envy. It is well beyond the scope of this book to explore the labyrinthine literature on this subject, so I will limit my discussion to dimensions that build on the theory discussed thus far and that have relevance for clinical practice.

Briefly, envy is the hatred one experiences toward an individual who possesses something desirable, arousing a sense of inferiority in the envious individual. When this occurs, it is not a matter of taking possession of this trait for oneself (which is characteristic of greed), but there is rather a need to *destroy* the envied trait, to spoil it so it no longer generates feelings of inferiority. (If something is ruined, it cannot provoke envy.) Given how unbearable it is for this object to possess this special trait, the urge to ruin it can be relentless, even if what is being attacked could be beneficial to the envious person. How might envy manifest itself?

As discussed previously, a good object can become persecutory during moments of withholding or absence. Ordinarily, even when the good object is not present, the "memory" of its existence remains (on a visceral, sensory level), and satisfaction can still be experienced when it returns and attends to the child. However, in some instances, when the child is overwhelmed by feelings of distress and hostility, the "goodness" of the object will not be experienced as such, but rather hatred can develop toward its giving, life-promoting abilities. When the good object attempts to lovingly interact with the child, the latter may feel this object's presence is contingent, short-lived, and predicated on its goodwill, well outside the child's control. This can generate re-

---

[8] This adaptation of the original lines was rendered by Klein. The source reads, "Certes, thanne is Envye the worste synne that is. For soothly, alle othere synnes been somtyme oonly agayns o special vertu, / but certes Envye is agayns alle vertues and agayns alle goodnesses" (Chaucer 1387–1400/2000) (Fragment X, Group I, 488–9) (p. 285).

sentiment in the child, who might act aggressively toward the purported good object, whose (usually) affiliative traits come to be equated with something that needs to be attacked. Moments that should be containing generate further distress and dissatisfaction. In effect, signs of goodness are viewed through a persecutory lens, because there is experiential knowledge that as soon as the good object opts to leave, the child will be left in a terrible state. This may make it impossible to take in the good object as something integrating. Because envy seeks to destroy something life-giving, it has been termed "the definitive version of the death drive" (Kristeva 2001, p. 95).

In short, as a derivative of anti-life forces, envy may represent a particular way in which aggressive urges can be overexpressed. It is, fundamentally, a *difficulty in experiencing the good object as good*. This can be viewed as existing on a spectrum for all of us, as opposed to something only present in a select few. We all feel unsettled at times, and what it takes for someone to reach and help us will vary between individuals and from one moment to the next. Similarly, we can think of some children who are much more easily soothed than others, promptly taking the bottle and being rocked to sleep. Others, however, may require much more attention and active caregiving, until the good object's abilities are experienced as intended.

Of course, no one can be fully under the aegis of hatefulness, because this would not be compatible with life. Even within the notion of envy there is a flicker of something loving because envy is predicated on the idea that good can be recognized as an active force in the world, even if it generates hatred. In some ways, it is the *good* of the world that has kept the individual alive and able to go on hating. Thus, the envious person is more in touch with and supported by something good and life-sustaining than one might wish to recognize.

Along these lines, Klein recognized that destructive urges exist alongside affiliative ones, with individual factors determining to what extent one may dominate at any given time.[9] (Klein conceptualized *gratitude*—a derivative of the life instinct—as the antithesis of envy.) This is critical in navigating the paranoid-schizoid position, as the child negotiates the presence of satisfying and frustrating objects, ideally consolidating ego integrity through enough "good" experiences to mitigate the pull toward unintegration caused by the "bad" ones. Klein stated, "Together with happy experiences, unavoidable

---

[9] Klein theorized that envy is an intrinsic force, operating from the first stages of life. As noted by Feldman and De Paola (1994), "According to Klein, and coherent with her view that envy is an innate (feeling/impulse) phenomenon, envy is present and active from birth as a direct expression of the death instinct, and is independent of any post-natal occurrence" (p. 223).

grievances reinforce the innate conflict between love and hate [...] and result in the feeling that a good and a bad breast exist. As a consequence, early emotional life is characterized by a sense of losing and regaining the good object" (Klein 1957/1975, p. 180).

Through repeated instances of gratification and frustration, the good object and its functions are internalized, as long as the deprivations are not too frequent or distressing. In an earlier work, Klein summarized this developmental process: "[A]ny such step in integration can only come about if [...] love towards the object predominates over the destructive impulses (ultimately the life instinct over the death instinct). The ego's tendency to integrate itself can, therefore, I think, be considered as an expression of the life instinct" (Klein 1952/1975, p. 65).

Envy can be present in the clinical setting as well. Attempts to provide a healing and supportive presence to patients might generate envy toward the therapist for possessing such affiliative capacities. Efforts to belittle and spoil the therapist's abilities can take place, lest the patient be consumed by envious feelings. (This can be particularly prominent in patients with narcissistic disorders because they can feel diminished or threatened by someone else's talents or creativity.) Such a dynamic can preclude establishment of a working alliance and limit therapeutic gain. It is better for envy-filled patients to suffer a *worsening* in symptoms than to allow their therapists the satisfaction of having been helpful.

Again, just as envious children may be unwittingly scaffolded by and in touch with the hated goodness more than they might realize, a patient coming to treatment to devalue the therapist is *still coming* to a setting that is predicated on understanding and healing. Thus, such patients are engaging with a potentially helpful person, putting themselves in a place where they could be reached, as much as hostility is at the forefront. We can imagine that tremendous pain and anxiety reside behind their defensive walls. Klein believed in the possibility of mitigating envy through continued therapeutic work. As Rustin and Rustin (2017) pointed out,

> Klein's tolerant and exploratory attitude enabled her patients to feel relief: envy could be contained and rendered knowable and in consequence become a less dangerous emotion, mitigated by feelings of gratitude for pain that had been understood. (...) Her hope for her patients is the re-integration of split-off, often destructive aspects of the self, the awareness of which initially causes shock, depression and anxiety but which, if held on to, can expand and strengthen the personality. (p. 116)

It is on this note that I will transition to discussing Bion. After presenting his views on learning and thinking, I will return to the concept of envy to outline how he approached the topic.

Bion

Wilfred Bion was a British-Indian psychoanalyst who was greatly influenced by the works of Klein, expanding on several of her concepts. Drawing from his own dreadful experiences in World War I (as developed in the book *The Long Week-End* [Bion 1982/2018]) and from his work with patients with psychosis, Bion wrote extensively on the interpersonal nature of thinking and emotional processing.

Among his key concepts are what Bion termed the "beta" and "alpha" elements or functions. He described beta-elements as "sense-impressions related to an emotional experience" (Bion 1962a, p. 17), which can be seen as unprocessed bits of information that keep one in touch with rawer versions of reality. We can imagine those hard-to-describe feelings of unease, restlessness, and dread as versions of beta-elements. We do not like feeling this way and try to come up with explanations that soothe our unsettled minds. Alternatively, we might try to induce the same feelings in *someone else*, ridding ourselves of them or at least sharing the burden. A distressed child will interact in such a way as to induce the caregiver to "feel" the distress as well, to take in the projected beta-elements, as it were. It is the caregiver's "alpha-function" that allows for these elements to be taken in and transformed (into alpha-elements), turning a raw and visceral feeling into something that can be thought about and contained. The child experiences this interaction as one in which the self's tormented inner state has been safely accessed and understood, leading to relief as opposed to mutual disintegration. This is in line with projective identification serving a communicative function. The child projects beta-elements into the caregiver, and the latter turns the sense impressions into something that can be lived through and learned from. As Bion stated, "Projective identification makes it possible for him to investigate his own feelings in a personality powerful enough to contain them" (Bion 1959, p. 314). This forms the basis for fostering a sense of curiosity about one's internal state, which has become less toxic and more knowable as a result of the caregiver's alpha-function. Such an instance of dyadic attunement and processing can be termed a *container-contained link* (Bion 1962a). The child (contained) projects into the caregiver or parent (container), who handles the projection in a loving and reassuring manner. This imbues a very distressing, raw emotion with meaning, permitting the child to further psychic development as a result. This is the crux of what Bion termed the "K Link" (K standing for "knowledge"), a search for truth and a desire to learn from experience, a tendency that has its roots in these very early interactions. Bion noted that

> the infant projects a part of its psyche, namely its bad feelings, into a good breast.(...)During their sojourn in the good breast they are felt to have been modified in such a way that the object that is re-introjected has become tol-

erable to the infant's psyche. (...) The earliest and most primitive manifestation of K occurs in the relationship between mother and infant. As a part
object relationship it may be stated as a relationship between mouth and
breast. (Bion 1962a, p. 90)

When such a model is the default, a child develops without needing to
resort to more extreme forms of interacting when dealing with uncertainty
because the good object (which has shown that distress can be dealt with benignly) will be internalized and help guide the individual through life as an
integrating presence. Life will be approached with openness, as something
of great possibility and excitement. The unknown is endowed with the potential for growth. This internalized function allows an individual to cultivate a thinking apparatus capable of processing and modifying internal
states as they emerge, without the need to get rid of them forcefully. Sitting
with uncertainty is not felt to be disintegrating. So, what happens when such
capacities are *not* fostered?

The alternative to thought modification is what can be termed "thought
evasion." For this to become the default in one's life, we can imagine that
containment by an attuned caregiver was mostly lacking in early interactions, making it difficult to process and integrate the vicissitudes of one's inner world into a consolidated sense of self. One can think of a child who is
feeling uncomfortable or scared and is met by an object's intolerance and
imperviousness to taking in the projections.[10] The child is left with the same
distressing beta-elements as before but now with the *added* dimension of
feeling alone with such difficult emotions, which can become terribly overwhelming and fill the child with a "nameless dread" (Bion 1962b, p. 309)
that threatens one with psychic disintegration. What the child feels is unwelcome, cannot be understood, and needs to be handled without any assistance from one's closest objects.

Such templates can be reinforced in a number of ways during development. For instance, a child innocently asks a question to which the narcis-
sistically fragile parent does not know the answer. Instead of the parent's
welcoming the child's curiosity and maybe seeing it as a fun opportunity for
both of them to learn something together, the parent is overtaken by the
danger of being seen as ignorant and is in effect threatened by the child's
mind. To deal with this, the parent says, "Hey, did you hear that question?
What a stupid kid. *Anyone* would know the answer to *that*. Go look it up, and
you'll see how obvious the answer is. Then you can come back and tell me
what you learned. I knew that at a much younger age than *you*." The child

---

[10] Skogstad (2013) used the term *impenetrable object* for such caregiver models.

will hardly be inspired to ever ask the parent a question again but will likely feel tremendous shame and confusion. Bion stated, "Denial of the use of this mechanism [of projective identification], [...] by the refusal of the mother to serve as a repository for the infant's feelings [...] leads to a destruction of the link between infant and breast and consequently to a severe disorder of the impulse to be curious on which all learning depends" (Bion 1959, p. 314).

The child will view the self's inner state, as confusing as it may be, as something that *cannot* be taken in by those in a position to provide integration and understanding. In the thought-modification model (facilitated by the caregiver's alpha-function), uncertainty provides the exciting prospect of learning and growth. If containment is lacking, uncertainty may pose a threat to psychic integrity. The child's unprocessed inner experiences will not be suitable for modification (because modeling did not occur); rather, they will be suitable only for immediate evacuation, lest they cause further disturbance. Bion said, "What should be a thought [...] becomes a bad object, indistinguishable from a thing-in-itself, fit only for evacuation. Consequently the development of an apparatus for thinking is disturbed. (...) The crux lies in the decision between modification and evasion of frustration" (Bion 1962b, p. 307).

There is little recourse left to the child but to find increasingly forceful modes of ridding the self of negative feelings. This may come at a great cost to psychic development because the child's internal world is impoverished by the incessant projection of unprocessed psychic elements. Doing so might bring some modicum of inner quiescence, but it also requires sacrificing one's curiosity and expression of creative gestures. A stultification or pseudo-maturation can occur, predicated on the impossibility that any further growth could take place. Bion powerfully commented,

> [R]refusal of the mother to serve as a repository for the infant's feelings [leads to] a destruction of the link. (...) Feelings of hatred are thereupon directed against all emotions. (...) It is a short step from hatred of the emotions to hatred of life itself. (...) [T]his hatred results in a resort to projective identification of all the perceptual apparatus including the embryonic thought which forms a link between sense impressions and consciousness. (Bion 1959, p. 314)

This hatred toward emotions and thinking is the crux of what Bion aptly called "−K" (minus K—the counterpart of the K Link) (Bion 1962a). In some cases, there may be "the assumption of omniscience as a substitute for learning from experience by the aid of thoughts and thinking" (Bion 1962b, p. 308). We can understand omniscience as a defense against the terror posed by uncertainty, which can leave one feeling exposed and filled with a dread that is impossible to process in more measured ways. The lesson learned from early life is that situations generating uncertainty need to be avoided at all costs, especially because no one will be able to help. As a solution to relying on the unpredictable minds of others or to needing to think about one's own internal experience, knowledge becomes ready-made and immutable.

Finally, I will return briefly to the concept of envy (which, again, we should conceptualize as difficulty in experiencing the good object as good because of the child's being overwhelmed by hostile or aggressive feelings). In this section on Bion, I posit that lack of containment can lead to the child's feeling replete with unprocessed dread, internalizing an object relationship that furthers confusion and pain rather than one that lessens them. This may be due to limitations in the caregiver, but as mentioned with envy, it may also be informed by constitutional factors in the child that make the child more demanding and harder to appease. Although the caregiving being provided might have been sufficiently contingent in more typical situations, a child's temperamental traits may be such that containment can prove extremely challenging. If contact is not effected to mitigate the child's distress, the end result is the reinforcement of a misattuned internal object. Bion stated,

> [The] infant is overwhelmed with hatred and envy of the mother's ability to retain a comfortable state of mind although experiencing the infant's feelings. This was clearly brought out by a patient who insisted that I must go through it with him, but was filled with hate when he felt I was able to do so without a breakdown. (…) Attacks on the link, therefore, are synonymous with attacks on the analyst's, and originally the mother's, peace of mind. (…) [P]eace of mind becomes hostile indifference. (Bion 1959, p. 313)

When an individual is filled with hateful feelings, reaching the part of that individual's mind that is capable of affiliative connection and growth is challenging. The guiding principle of the internal world will be one of antidevelopment forces supervening over those of curiosity, learning, and healthy development, whether driven by intrinsic factors in the child or by faults in caregiving (or what is most likely a combination). In such a state, "−K" is in the ascendant. Hatred toward one's own mind, particularly the part of it capable of actually being reached and helped by another, will compete with the desire to cultivate something more loving and connected with others. This is an important conceptual point because the individual may internalize an envy- and hate-filled object relationship template alongside one in which some contact *is* possible. In subsequent interactions (including in therapy), there can be shifts between moments of relatedness and a strong shutting down of such a dynamic. What can be appreciated in this moment is that connectedness feels risky and that this feeling activates the "hate-filled" internal object to punitively and enviously attack these gossamer links the individual was tentatively forging with another person. What has been termed the "ego-destructive superego" (Bion 1959, p. 314) represents this introject seeking to denude the ego of its qualities, reacting with hostility at any movement on the part of the individual toward greater connectedness and growth. We can see corollaries of this in adult life, wherein achieving success (or even making positive or healthy changes) may be verboten because of an internal object that is intolerant of psychic development, seeking to keep the individual in a state of nonevolving paralysis, unable to think or to be reached.

Attachment Schema

Although not the primary theoretical orientation of this book, I will provide a brief outline of the different types of attachment schema because these are established largely within the first year of life and will be referred to in my discussion of the neurosciences. There are also important parallels with aspects of object relations theory, upon which I will elaborate later in this chapter.

Attachment research in humans evolved from scientific findings in the field of ethology produced by scientists including Nikolaas Tinbergen, Harry Harlow, and Konrad Lorenz. John Bowlby expanded on the importance of the attachment system in human development (Bowlby 1969, 1973, 1980; see also Holmes 2014). He described how the set goal of this system is "felt security" (as opposed to physical distance regulation). In childhood development, there is a dynamic balance between attachment and exploration behaviors, with the mediating influence of fear. The greater the felt security, the more the child is able to maintain some physical distance from the caregiver and explore the environment. As children negotiate this, they also learn what behaviors on their part may draw their caregivers in (e.g., smiling, crying, bodily forms of expression). Through these behaviors, children detect regularities ("if-then"), with contingencies becoming *expectancies* about how the child's behaviors will affect those of the caregiver. For Bowlby, a typical response sequence to object separation was 1) protest (e.g., signs of anger, following the caregiver, crying loudly); 2) despair and withdrawal, with increased hopelessness about the caregiver's return, a decrease in physical movements, and a disengagement from people in the environment; and 3) detachment, wherein the child no longer rejects alternative caregivers and may show a lack of joy at the return of the caregiver who originally departed. (For some children, this detachment may alternate with clinging behaviors and a fear that the caregiver might leave again.) For a vivid depiction of this response sequence, readers are referred to the videos by James and Joyce Robertson from the series titled *Young Children in Brief Separation*. The investigators longitudinally followed and depicted children's behavioral and affective reactions to being separated from their caregivers, as well as the children's responses upon being reunited with them.

Developmental psychologist Mary Ainsworth devised a series of brief, "minuscule separations" in young children (typically around 52 weeks of age) (Ainsworth and Bell 1970; Ainsworth and Wittig 1969).[11] These experiments (termed "the Strange Situation") lasted roughly 20 minutes, broken into eight distinct steps. In them, Ainsworth described the interplay between the attachment and exploration systems, mediated by the infant's use of the mother as a "secure base" from which to explore. The steps were as follows:

Step 1: Parent and infant are introduced to the experimental room.

Step 2: Parent and infant are alone. Parent does not participate while infant explores.

Step 3: Stranger enters, converses with parent, then approaches infant. Parent leaves inconspicuously.

Step 4: First separation episode. Stranger's behavior is geared to that of the infant. If the child is engaged in play, Stranger is nonparticipant. If the child is inactive, Stranger tries to engage the child with toys. If the child is distressed, Stranger tries to provide distraction or comfort.

Step 5: First reunion episode. Parent greets and comforts infant (while Stranger exits the room), then leaves again.

Step 6: Second separation episode. Infant is left alone.

Step 7: Continuation of second separation episode. Stranger enters and gears behavior to that of infant (similar to what was described in Step 4).

Step 8: Second reunion episode. Parent enters, greets and picks up infant; Stranger leaves inconspicuously.

Perhaps unsurprisingly, exploration peaked when the child was alone with the mother (Step 2) and decreased as subsequent steps took place. Prox-

---

[11] Strange Situation paradigms have been investigated in ages typically varying from 9 months to 2 years. The mobility component (e.g., play, exploration, and proximity-seeking) is crucial in gauging a child's response to separation from the caregiver. In DSM-5-TR, conditions related to attachment (under "Trauma- and Stressor-Related Disorders") include reactive attachment disorder and disinhibited social engagement disorder (American Psychiatric Association 2022). The text mentions that these conditions should not be diagnosed before children are able to form selective attachments, further stating, "For this reason, the child must have a developmental age of at least 9 months" (American Psychiatric Association 2022, pp. 296, 299).

imity-seeking behaviors increased from the initial step through the last, as caregiver availability was shown to be at risk. Bottom line: as attachment system activation increases, exploration system activation *decreases*. In her initial descriptions of the Strange Situation, Ainsworth characterized three behavioral response styles in young children.

- Secure attachment (type B): Securely attached children use the mother as a safe base from which to explore their environment. Upon separation from the mother, the child shows distress. The child is avoidant of the stranger when the two are alone but shows friendliness when the mother is present. During the reunion episodes, the child is happy with the mother's return.
- Insecure attachment—anxious avoidant (type A): This child exhibits a lack of confidence in the caregiver's availability, downregulating emotional arousal when the caregiver is present *or* absent. During separation, the child shows no clear sign of distress. When alone with the stranger, the child plays normally. When the mother returns, the child shows little interest.
- Insecure attachment—anxious ambivalent/resistant (type C): In this attachment type, children *up*regulate or exaggerate their affective responses, trying to secure the caregiver's attention. During separation, the child shows signs of being intensely distressed. When alone with the stranger, the child avoids or seems affrighted by this individual. When the mother returns, the child shows ambivalence, approaching her but resisting contact, even pushing her away at times. This child, compared with the other two types, exhibits less exploratory behavior.

The degree to which a child feels secure about caregiver availability is a critical consideration when one is contrasting these attachment types. In type B, there is enough of a basic sense of safety that the child can endure moments of uncertainty and separation without becoming too activated or shutting down. When the mother returns, the child is able to reengage without having been overly affected by her absence. In types A and C, caregiver presence and responsiveness are not assumed; the child adopts strategies to negotiate the perceived unresponsiveness of the attachment figure by decreasing or heightening affect, respectively.

Ainsworth later correlated certain behavioral response patterns in children with particular parenting styles (Ainsworth et al. 1978). For children who had inconsistent, underinvolved, or unreliable caregiving, behavioral strategies de-emphasized exploration and prioritized attachment. If a caregiver was overbearing, overly intrusive, or rebuffing of attachment behaviors, the child might adopt avoidance as a strategy to shut down engagement.

In addition to the three attachment styles described previously, Mary Main (one of Ainsworth's students) later added a fourth, termed *disorganized/disoriented* (type D) (Main and Hesse 1990; Main and Solomon 1990). This type may be observed in children with chaotic or traumatizing upbringings under frightening, unpredictable caregivers. In such conditions, the child does not develop coherent attachment behaviors. Rather, there is a breakdown in any organized attempt to deal with distress because the child may be hard wired to look to a damaging object in search of safety. Notably, the resulting confusion and disorientation may be reflected in the child's behaviors (e.g., freezing or staying still, alternating movements toward and away from the caregiver, walking backward toward the caregiver). These contradictory behaviors suggest that both alarm and security are competing to form the organizing lens through which the caregiver is seen.

Critically, there is evidence that certain attachment styles can be *perpetuated into one's adulthood* (Critchfield and Benjamin 2008), making them very relevant for work with adult patients. Akin to how a child's internalized object relationships are formed through encoding of experiences with others in early development, Bowlby described "representational models" or "internal working models" that become consolidated in the child and orient how that individual interacts with others throughout life. For a developing child, such models would be determined by how caregivers were expected to respond (or not), as well as by the child's sense of "how acceptable or unacceptable he himself is in the eyes of his attachment figures" (Bowlby 1973, p. 203). He compared the establishment of working models with the process of introjecting a good or bad object, which takes place in tandem with internalization of a child's perceived "self-image" (Bowlby 1973, p. 204). He also emphasized how selection of certain environments by an individual can be a way of reinforcing internalized modes of relating in accordance with working models.

One can draw parallels between these concepts and object relations theory, including how transference dynamics can inform us about patients' attachment styles (particularly germane if childhood patterns have persisted into adulthood). For instance, the Strange Situation paradigm may be invoked when thinking about the implications of the frame in therapy (e.g., ending a session, the ensuing break, and being "reunited" with the therapist in the next session). How the object is perceived and negotiated by the patient can be linked with different attachment types, as I will briefly outline.

- Within sessions, during breaks, and upon returning, the patient's need for the therapist or object is disavowed or de-emphasized. Even if on some level the patient wants or needs the object to be organizing and attuned, such an acknowledgment is a recognition of vulnerability and dependence, incurring the possibility of being dropped. As such, connectedness is shut down, and the therapist is devalued so as not to be necessary. We could compare this form of response to attachment type A (avoidant).

- Session endings and breaks are met by the patient with an upregulation of affect. For a child with type C attachment, separation was *so* destabilizing that turning to extreme measures to guarantee proximity might have been the only strategy available. Patients may resort to similarly pressurized methods around the fringes of sessions, such as making doorknob suicidal statements, demanding for time to be extended or for contact between sessions to be allowed, or asking for medications after time is up (perhaps to have something "concrete" to take with them to narrow the gap). I had a patient who would leave voice messages on my answering machine between sessions, though he sometimes had nothing to say (leaving me puzzled by the "silent" voice message). He told me he frequently did this just to hear my voice on the recording, without which our time apart could feel unbearable. He said he needed reassurance I was still alive and had not suddenly quit my job and moved elsewhere.

- A patient with a good, containing internal object can maintain a sense of self and therapist as whole objects during moments of separation *without* experiencing despair or indifference. The working model of a secure relationship allows for continued exploration to take place upon reuniting. In other words, the gaps between sessions do not diminish the patient's confidence in the availability and value of the therapist. This is akin to a secure attachment style.

- In some cases, there may be an almost obsessive obedience to the parameters we outline, with patients never arriving late or canceling a session. In cases of early adversity and introjection of a bad, persecuting object, patients may worry about what it might take for us to "become" this monstrous object that demands absolute obedience. The fact that these patients keep coming back suggests *some* desire for contact, yet it is confused by the internal working model directing them to be fearful of that same object to which they are drawn (as described earlier, feelings of alarm and security are competing). Patients may begin sessions with great reticence, carefully gauging the type of object to which they have returned. They might need to "feel us out" by minimizing talk and heightening awareness, watching for nods, smiles, and other signs "confirming" we are safe and receptive objects. In effect, patients do not take our availability and consistency for granted. Rather, there is a need to reaffirm these qualities constantly, lest the patients be left at the mercy of a destructive object they cannot control. This mode of relating is suggestive of a disorganized attachment style.

The theoretical base presented in this chapter will help ground readers in the clinical vignettes to follow. Namely, I will outline how early life templates may be repeated in clinical encounters, drawing particular attention to transference-countertransference dynamics.

KEY POINTS

- A child's early environment and objects will have a critical role in consolidating one's sense of self and others.

- A facilitative environment, in the presence of a "good-enough" caregiver, will help children discover the scope and limitations of their abilities. This will be important when navigating the challenges of the Oedipal situation.

- During the pre-Oedipal period, objects are viewed as all-good and all-bad, with a greater nuance gradually being afforded to objects as positive, affirming experiences outweigh the frustrating, depriving ones.

- If adversity is the norm, split-object models may persist, with a narrowing of one's sense of self and others, limiting curiosity and the ability to learn from experience.

- Dimensions of attachment theory, including types of governing schema (secure, insecure, disorganized) and the concept of "internal working models," have important correlations with the internalization of object relationship templates that takes place in childhood.

References

Ainsworth MD, Bell SM: Attachment, exploration, and separation: illustrated by the behavior of one-year-olds in a strange situation. Child Dev 41(1):49–67, 1970 5490680

Ainsworth M, Wittig B: Attachment and exploratory behavior of one-year-olds in a strange situation, in Determinants of Infant Behavior, Vol 4. Edited by Foss B. London, Methuen, 1969, pp 111–136

Ainsworth M, Blehar M, Waters E, Wall S: Patterns of Attachment: A Psychological Study of the Strange Situation. Hillsdale, NJ, Erlbaum, 1978

American Psychiatric Association: Diagnostic and Statistical Manual of Mental Disorders, 5th Edition, Text Revision. Washington, DC, American Psychiatric Association, 2022

Bandura A: Influence of model's reinforcement contingencies on the acquisition of imitative responses. J Pers Soc Psychol 1:589–595, 1965 14300234

Bandura A, Ross D, Ross SA: Imitation of film-mediated aggressive models. J Abnorm Soc Psychol 66:3–11, 1963 13966304

Belsky J: Variation in susceptibility to environmental influence: an evolutionary argument. Psychol Inq 8:182–186, 1997

Belsky J, Bakermans-Kranenburg MJ, Van IJzendoorn MH: For better and for worse: differential susceptibility to environmental influences. Curr Dir Psychol Sci 16:300–304, 2007

Belsky J, Jonassaint C, Pluess M, et al: Vulnerability genes or plasticity genes? Mol Psychiatry 14(8):746–754, 2009 19455150

Bion W: Attacks on linking. Int J Psychoanal 40:308–315, 1959

Bion W: Learning From Experience. London, Karnac, 1962a

Bion WR: The psycho-analytic study of thinking: a theory of thinking. Int J Psychoanal 43:306–310, 1962b 13968380

Bion W: Elements of Psychoanalysis (1963). Oxford, UK, Routledge, 2018

Bion W: The Long Week-End (1982). Oxford, UK, Routledge, 2018

Blos P: The second individuation process of adolescence. Psychoanal Study Child 22:162–186, 1967 5590064

Bowlby J: Attachment and Loss, Vol 1: Attachment. London, Hogarth Press and the Institute of Psycho-Analysis, 1969

Bowlby J: Attachment and Loss, Vol 2: Separation, Anxiety and Anger. London, Hogarth Press and the Institute of Psycho-Analysis, 1973

Bowlby J: Attachment and Loss, Vol 3: Loss, Sadness and Depression. London, Hogarth Press and the Institute of Psycho-Analysis, 1980

Chaucer G: The parson's tale, in The Canterbury Tales (1387–1400). Edited by Benson L. Boston, MA, Houghton Mifflin, 2000, pp 269–310

Chugani HT, Behen ME, Muzik O, et al: Local brain functional activity following early deprivation: a study of postinstitutionalized Romanian orphans. Neuroimage 14(6):1290–1301, 2001 11707085

Critchfield KL, Benjamin LS: Internalized representations of early interpersonal experience and adult relationships: a test of copy process theory in clinical and nonclinical settings. Psychiatry 71(1):71–92, 2008 18377207

Eluvathingal TJ, Chugani HT, Behen ME, et al: Abnormal brain connectivity in children after early severe socioemotional deprivation: a diffusion tensor imaging study. Pediatrics 117(6):2093–2100, 2006 16740852

Erikson E: Identity and the Life Cycle (1959). New York, WW Norton, 1980

Feldman E, De Paola H: An investigation into the psychoanalytic concept of envy. Int J Psychoanal 75 (Pt 2):217–234, 1994 8063480

Forcada-Guex M, Pierrehumbert B, Borghini A, et al: Early dyadic patterns of mother-infant interactions and outcomes of prematurity at 18 months. Pediatrics 118(1):e107–e114, 2006 16818525

Freud S: Three essays on the theory of sexuality (1905), in The Standard Edition of the Complete Psychological Works of Sigmund Freud, Vol 7. Translated and edited by Strachey J. London, Hogarth Press, 1953, pp 123–246

Freud S: Instincts and their vicissitudes (1915), in The Standard Edition of the Complete Psychological Works of Sigmund Freud, Vol 14. Translated and edited by Strachey J. London, Hogarth Press, 1957, pp 109–140

Freud S: Beyond the pleasure principle (1920), in The Standard Edition of the Complete Psychological Works of Sigmund Freud, Vol 18. Translated and edited by Strachey J. London, Hogarth Press, 1955, pp 1–64

Greenberg TM: Psychodynamic Perspectives on Aging and Illness. New York, Springer, 2009

Holmes J: John Bowlby and Attachment Theory, 2nd Edition. Makers of Modern Psychotherapy. Hove, East Sussex, UK, Routledge, 2014

Khan MM: The concept of cumulative trauma. Psychoanal Study Child 18:286–306, 1963 14147282

Klein M: Early development of conscience in the child (1933) in Love, Guilt and Reparation and Other Works 1921–1945 (The Writings of Melanie Klein), Vol 1. Edited by Money-Kyrle R. New York, Free Press, 1975, pp 248–257

Klein M: A contribution to the psychogenesis of manic depressive states (1935), in Love, Guilt and Reparation and Other Works 1921–1945 (The Writings of Melanie Klein), Vol 1. Edited by Money-Kyrle R. New York, Free Press, 1975, pp 262–289

Klein M: Notes on some schizoid mechanisms. Int J Psychoanal 27 (Pt 3–4):99–110, 1946 20261821

Klein M: Some theoretical conclusions regarding the emotional life of the infant (1952), in Envy and Gratitude and Other Works 1946–1963. Edited by Khan M. London, Hogarth Press, 1975, pp 61–93

Klein M: Envy and gratitude (1957), in Envy and Gratitude and Other Works 1946–1963. Edited by Khan M. London, Hogarth Press, 1975, pp 176–235

Klein M: On the development of mental functioning. Int J Psychoanal 39(2–4):84–90, 1958 13574941

Kristeva J: Melanie Klein. New York, Columbia University Press, 2001

Kumsta R, Kreppner J, Rutter M, et al: III. Deprivation-specific psychological patterns. Monogr Soc Res Child Dev 75(1):48–78, 2010 20500633

Kumsta R, Kreppner J, Kennedy M, et al: Psychological consequences of early global deprivation: an overview of findings from the English & Romanian Adoptees study. Eur Psychol 20:138–151, 2015

Mackes NK, Golm D, Sarkar S, et al: Early childhood deprivation is associated with alterations in adult brain structure despite subsequent environmental enrichment. Proc Natl Acad Sci USA 117(1):641–649, 2020 31907309

Main M, Hesse E: Parents' unresolved traumatic experiences are related to infant disorganized attachment status: is frightened and/or frightening parental behavior the linking mechanism? in Attachment in the Preschool Years: Theory, Research, and Intervention. Edited by Greenberg M, Cicchetti D, Cummings M. Chicago, IL, University of Chicago Press, 1990, pp 161–184

Main M, Solomon J: Procedures for identifying infants as disorganized/disoriented during the Ainsworth Strange Situation, in Attachment in the Preschool Years: Theory, Research, and Intervention. Edited by Greenberg M, Cicchetti D, Cummings M. Chicago, IL, University of Chicago Press, 1990, pp 121–160

Malatesta CZ, Culver C, Tesman JR, Shepard B: The development of emotion expression during the first two years of life. Monogr Soc Res Child Dev 54(1–2):1–104, discussion 105–136, 1989 2770755

Milne AA: Now We Are Six (1927). New York, Dutton Children's Books, 1988

Novick KK, Novick J: Postoedipal transformations: latency, adolescence, and pathogenesis. J Am Psychoanal Assoc 42(1):143–169, 1994 8182242

Quinodoz D: Growing Old: A Journey of Self-Discovery. Hove, East Sussex, UK, Routledge, 2010

Rustin M, Rustin M: Reading Klein. New Library of Psychoanalysis "Teaching" Series. Oxford, UK, Routledge, 2017

Rutter M, Kreppner J, Croft C, et al: Early adolescent outcomes of institutionally deprived and non-deprived adoptees: III: quasi-autism. J Child Psychol Psychiatry 48(12):1200–1207, 2007 18093025

Segal H: Introduction to the Work of Melanie Klein. Oxford, UK, Routledge, 1988

Shapiro G, Jaffe R, Kolevzon A: Normal child development, in Kaplan and Sadock's Comprehensive Textbook of Psychiatry. Edited by Sadock B, Sadock V, Ruiz P. Philadelphia, PA, Wolters Kluwer, 2017, pp 3351–3364

Skogstad W: Impervious and intrusive: the impenetrable object in transference and countertransference. Int J Psychoanal 94(2):221–238, 2013 23560900

Sorce J, Emde R, Campos J, Klinnert M: Maternal emotional signaling: its effect on the visual cliff behavior of 1-year-olds. Dev Psychol 21:195–200, 1985

Tarkovsky AA: Andrei Tarkovsky: A Cinema Prayer. New York, Criterion Collection, 2019

Vygotsky L: Mind in Society: The Development of Higher Psychological Processes. Cambridge, MA, Harvard University Press, 1978

Winnicott DW: Aggression and its roots (1939), in Deprivation and Delinquency. Edited by Winnicott C, Shepherd R, Davis M. New York, Routledge, 1964, pp 73–85

Winnicott DW: Transitional objects and transitional phenomena; a study of the first not-me possession. Int J Psychoanal 34(2):89–97, 1953 13061115

Winnicott DW: Primary maternal preoccupation (1956), in Through Pediatrics to Psycho-analysis. Edited by Khan M. New York, Routledge, 1992, pp 300–305

Winnicott DW: The capacity to be alone (1958), in The Maturational Processes and the Facilitating Environment. Edited by Khan M. London, Hogarth Press and the Institute of Psycho-Analysis, 1965, pp 29–36

Winnicott DW: The theory of the parent-infant relationship. Int J Psychoanal 41:585–595, 1960 13785877

Winnicott DW: Ego distortion in terms of true and false self (1960), in The Maturational Processes and the Facilitating Environment. Edited by Khan M. London, Hogarth Press and the Institute of Psycho-Analysis, 1965, pp 140–152

Winnicott DW: The use of an object. Int J Psychoanal 50:711–716, 1969

Developing a Sense of Self: Clinical

We should be so constituted that we can at any time be placed in a
different position without offering resistance or losing our heads.

Hermann Hesse (1943/2012, p. 82)

To CONSOLIDATE the material presented in Chapter 6 ("Developing a Sense of Self: Theory"), I will outline how these concepts can be applied to clinical encounters, both in psychotherapy and in acute care. In doing so, I will reinforce the utility of the object relations lens across settings, with particular emphasis on how paranoid-schizoid dynamics may be prominent during interactions in adult life. This can result from lack of sufficient environment and object scaffolding, necessary for an integrated and nuanced sense of self to develop. Governing object relationships may be narrowed in scope, and providers in clinical settings can feel tremendous pressure to reinforce early templates through projective identification.

Acute Care Settings

In quick-paced, higher-intensity settings such as the emergency department (ED), we may be more susceptible to identifying with our patients' internal objects because there is limited time to process what is taking place. Indeed, we might find ourselves unwittingly participating in reenactments, only reflecting on them *after* they have occurred.

These settings are at times the only resource thought to be available for patients with very complex psychosocial scenarios (e.g., experiencing homelessness, lack of support, concurrent substance use), situations that would ordinarily necessitate layered and stepwise interventions. However, adversity is often very much the norm for some of our patients, with the internalized object relations template being one of misattunement and rejection.[1] Given lack of nuanced object differentiation based on experiences of containment, splitting can predominate. As such, we may find ourselves under pressure to recapitulate the role of bad object (e.g., as the dispassionate provider who will drop or discharge the patient without anything being resolved) or live out the opposite end of the split—that of the idealized object. Importantly, this latter object is *not* exemplified by a thoughtful provider who outlines a road map for patients to slowly regain a more satisfying footing in their outside and internal worlds, with joint provider-patient participation. Rather, the idealized object is one that is all-resolving, one that does not force the patient to re-introject *anything* that is being pushed out. This idealized, part-object role we are cast in promises compensation for what was lacking early in life— an environment-object that is holistically and sensorially containing, one that provides food, quietness, warmth, and protection from undue stimuli. Aligned with this is my observation that many patients feel much safer in a locked emergency setting (when it is available) compared with something less re-strictive. Sometimes the walls do a much better job of providing a holding experience than our words ever could. We are sought not for our thinking capacity but for the physicality of the environment we offer. When soothing comes from our mechanical qualities, our mental prowess is unnecessary and unwelcome.[2]

When words *are* used, they are employed in evacuative ways, not in the service of fostering communication. If our minds do serve a function, it is as a receptacle for unprocessed projections (which should be kept in us, *not* modified through thinking and delivered back to patients). This may underlie the displeasure it causes some patients when they are expected to "repeat everything all over again." (For instance, in teaching hospitals, patients are interviewed, with varying levels of detail, two or three separate times.) For patients wishing to evacuate thought, the hope would be that once the problem was explained the first time, it would be "out there," contained concretely in

---

[1] The rates of traumatic histories in patients in EDs can be staggeringly high.

[2] This is something we might notice in therapy sessions as well. It can feel at times like patients come to be "held" for 50 minutes, not wishing to think at all. Transference may develop to the spatial and physical qualities of the office or therapist. The provider's mind can indeed become an intrusive presence interfering with sensory holding. In his article on the "transformational object," Christopher Bollas (1979) spoke to this use of the therapist by the patient, detailing how this fantasy can develop.

the words now etched into the provider's mind and *not* something that would need to be dealt with "again." (For instance, after asking a patient how it is we can help, we may be given the answer, "I just told you how I feel. *You're* the doctor. *You* do the work now.") If a different provider asks a repeat question after the patient has just gone through an interview, the anger can be palpable because the patient might feel that everything that has just been said has been dropped.[3] When one is wishing to evacuate tormenting psychic bits at all costs, it can be despairing to realize the problem is *not* "out there" but remains very much *inside* the patient's mind. The projection has failed, and a merciless re-introjection is forced on the patient, who might feel it is impossible to rid the self of these assailing beta-elements. A female patient self-presented to the emergency room and I was the first person to interview her. When I asked "What brought you in today?" she grabbed her head despairingly and screamed back, "I showed up, didn't I? Doesn't that tell you enough? You keep asking me all these questions, question after question, nonstop! Can't you shut up and do your job for once? I've *told* you *everything*!" It was evocative of a young child, confused and desperate, demanding her right to a caregiver who will scoop her up and comfort her, *without* pushing words onto her or forcing her to think in such a terrible and fragile moment. A child indeed only needs to show up; the caregiver's job is to do the rest, making the child feel at ease and contained. From her perspective, my question likely recapitulated the impingements of a demanding early environment because it might have seemed I was favoring my own agenda while disregarding her immediate distress tolerance and holding needs.[4]

When a provider is treated as an idealized object (i.e., one possessing *all* the solutions to a patient's struggles), *any* deviation from this projected role incurs the risk of being recast as the polar opposite—a depriving, persecutory object. As discussed, splitting may predominate in patients who suffered extensive early trauma, given the lack of a "good-enough" environment to consolidate whole-object perspectives. Colored by fantasy, part-object introjects can become quite extreme in nature, including the belief that a perfect object exists *somewhere*, the antithesis of the abusive one experienced in reality. Such a fantasy provides a modicum of self-comfort amid the terror of a chaotic surround. Echoes of this can be gleaned from one's treatment of inani-

---

[3] This is not to discount that there is very understandable frustration involved in having to repeat information several times, especially when one is feeling anxious and upset. I am rather emphasizing cases in which any kind of investigation or inquiry feels invasive.

[4] I have described elsewhere how acute care settings can prove retraumatizing, especially when there is very limited time to work with individual patients (Miller 2019).

mate objects, felt to carry the attributes of perfectly attuned caregivers. After all, a doll or stuffed animal 1) is always immediately available, 2) will never leave (even if treated aggressively), 3) always has a smile on its face, 4) is soft and comforting, 5) may be felt to understand the child better than any human has, and (perhaps most important) 6) is something utterly predictable and under the child's complete control.

For traumatized children with unstable rearing environments, the fantasy of the perfect object can be projected strongly into foster parents, who will experience great pressure to conform to these demands. If unable to, they may give the child up to another family or to a group home, aligning with the opposite split-object role, that of an uncaring and abandoning object, the counterpoint to the perfect one conjured up.

Later in life, the fury of the "perfect object" fantasy can come storming into the clinical encounter, with the provider being viewed as dividend for the abuse the patient sustained throughout life. If the provider is unable to meet the demands for such all-encompassing solutions (which seems inevitable), the provider can become equated with the abandoning, misattuned object. In such instances, patients might disengage completely, actively ensuring the provider will be experienced as someone who cannot reach them, reinforcing the all-bad, split-object projection.

A variation on the wish for an idealized object experience can be observed in suicidal patients who present to the emergency room stating they are coming to us as their "last hope." We are told that any chance of being salvaged is on our shoulders because they have otherwise "given up on life." This is also not uncommon in individuals who have suffered extensive adversity. Through projective identification, we may indeed feel we *are* their only chance. This is further complicated by our attempts to remain in a thinking mode, as we ponder inconsistencies in the narrative (for instance, reading in the chart that the patient had the same presentation on multiple occasions). Our attempts to retain such "whole-object" status should not obscure our empathic concern for *why we need to be viewed as messianic objects* that will take the patient's rock-bottom despair at face value. Patients might exert such molding pressures on providers as a way of confirming that *goodness actually exists* in the world. To this end, patients can make themselves more pitiful, ill-appearing, or helpless—extreme but *necessary* ways of proving, through our response, that there is a counterpoint to the all-bad object (an entity with which the patient may have much greater familiarity and whose existence needs no further proof). As such, even when we are being split off as an idealized object and noting patients' resistance to any self-advocacy, embedded in this dynamic is the hope that somewhere, in some form, *someone* is invested in keeping them alive.

Clinical Vignettes

To illustrate some of the concepts outlined so far, I will now present two vignettes from my work in the psychiatric emergency services.

Vignette 1

Mr. A was a 40-year-old man with chronic substance use and a history of early trauma who had been in a number of unsatisfactory living environments (mainly recovery homes) in recent weeks. He presented to the ED after being asked to leave his most recent transitional housing because of an altercation with a peer. He seemed quite irritable and withdrawn, making minimal eye contact with me during my assessment. As the interview progressed, he did show moments of relaxation, though these were immediately followed by a tensing of the body, a hostile stare, and suspicious interrogation of my motives for asking him questions, with statements such as "You're just going to discharge me without offering me any help, aren't you? Then just *do* it!" We were up against a very hostile template. I reassured him of my commitment to his well-being and that I would endeavor to find a treatment option he deemed appropriate. I acquiesced to his (very reasonable) requests for medications to assist with substance withdrawal. He seemed surprised by this and even cracked a smile at the end of the interview. I left the interview area to work on disposition options, and after some time, he called me back. He was worked up and seemed ready for a fight. He said, "You have bad news.…I just know it. You're going to discharge me. You fucking doctors.…You're all the same. Fucking useless."

Feeling very tense, I asked him to have a seat so we could talk, which he did. He continued to mumble angrily to himself. I said, "I actually have some good news. We're working on placement at a co-occurring disorders unit [i.e., one that would address psychiatric and substance use concerns, which was what he had hoped for] and we're going to send the paperwork over there for approval."

Seemingly stunned, he looked down and grabbed his head with both hands. He appeared tortured by what was taking place inside his mind, as though he wished to physically *push out* something that was invading him. As he rocked back and forth in a state of agitation, he enunciated in an angrily confused way, "That…sounds…GREAT!" It was an affront to the cleanness of the split. Even if we did have a moment of connectedness during the initial interview, my brief physical absence was enough time for his sadistic internal objects to take hold once more, recasting me as a depriving, all-bad object who was not to be trusted. When I reaffirmed my place as a potentially more benign object (presenting him with a desirable treatment plan), this was terribly confusing, leading to an unbearable cognitive dissonance. The only way to restore any psychic balance would be to change his perception of reality, forcing the projection to hold.[5] He looked up at me from his chair and shouted, "You're LYING!!" He refused to speak any further and demanded to be discharged.

Vignette 2

Mr. B was a 50-year-old man I saw for an intake in my outpatient clinic. He had struggled with depression for many years. He shared with me the difficulties he experienced during his upbringing, particularly how inconsistently available his parents had been. (They were divorced by the time he was born.) He described being frequently "shunted" from one parent to the other, as though he were a problem to be rid of, with neither assuming any lasting responsibility for his well-being. He frequently became hopeful that this pattern would change and that one of his parents would finally "adopt [him] for good," yet this always led to disappointment and a renewed sense of abandonment when the other parent was summoned to take him away again. A variation of this cycle was lived out by us over the course of 2 days.

We spent a fair amount of time on the intake, discussing his concerns about the actual benefits of engaging in psychiatric treatment. I noticed myself trying very hard to maintain contact with the part of him that thought I *could* help, conjuring the mental image of a rope slowly slipping away from my grip, though I still held on tightly. After 60 very tense minutes, he produced a tentative smile, stating he felt hopeful for the first time in many years. We agreed we would meet again in a week to continue discussing our treatment goals and how best to approach them.

The next day, I was working in the ED. The resident had just seen a patient on her own and wanted to present the case to me so we could develop a treatment plan. The resident told me she felt concerned about how tearful and despondent the patient had been during the interview. The patient said he had always felt lost and alone, unworthy of being understood or cared for by anyone. He said his despair was so immense that only immediate hospitalization could address it. The resident had experienced a lot of tension in the room, feeling like something burdensome was being pushed into her. She left the evaluation feeling like the lone bearer of all responsibility for the patient's well-being and potential for improvement.

When the resident and I walked to the interview room to talk to the patient, it was a most extraordinary moment. It was Mr. B. He had his head low-

---

[5] As Ogden (1979) said, "Reality that is not useful in confirming a projection is treated as if it did not exist" (p. 360).

ered and was quite tearful. That is, until he raised his eyes and saw me. The look he gave me was one of stunned outrage, as though he had been confronted with something he had gone to great lengths to eliminate from his awareness. He begrudgingly answered my questions in a curt, irritated manner. The resident was clearly confused, as though what she was witnessing with Mr. B did not align at all with her initial impressions of him. I talked to Mr. B:

> T: We just met yesterday and came up with a plan to talk next week.
> P: I know....I felt good yesterday....Then I started doubting the whole thing after I left.
> T: You doubted the whole thing.
> P: I doubted *you*. You wanted us *both* to be thinking about this together. That sounded good in theory, but the more I thought about it, the less I liked it.
> T: It seemed to sound good in practice, too. You brought so much of yourself into our talk yesterday and left seeming more optimistic despite all the doubts you had about whether I could help.
> P: I *am* opti—I mean, I *was* optimistic....Then it just seemed like too much work. I'd rather just get admitted.
> T: It's hard to stay in that place where you believe in both *my* wish to help you and in *your own* feeling that what you have to say is something to be listened to and thought about with great care. You may figure I'll just drop you, like others have done to you in the past, and you'll need to find someone else to treat you. You re-created that in a way by seeing me yesterday and then coming here today to see someone different. Although it all feels so fragile, I imagine you have *some* hope that we could work together and that something more transformative could happen over time. If we hold onto that, the more concrete and short-lived solution of being hospitalized may not be necessary.
> P: (He begins crying again, slowly nodding his head as he brushes away tears.) Yes....There's so much I've wanted to share, for so long....I actually am a special person with...Whatever....Just leave me alone for a bit, please.

I exited the interview room with the resident, who wondered what led Mr. B to shift so much from how he was at first. My sense of the situation was that he had only briefly been able to come into contact with the idea of relatedness and continuity, which faded away after he left my office. The fickle, abandoning internal object then asserted its influence, reminding him others were unreliable and would ultimately drop him, no matter how welcoming they might seem. (He knew this never lasted.) By coming to the emergency room to speak to someone else, he turned me *into* an object that was only available intermittently, on my own terms. Through my absence, I was an active participant in this traumatizing reenactment.

The part of him that had engaged in our previous session, a part capable of relating to others and investing in his own growth, had not been held onto after he left the office. Rather, it was split off and projected out. (The resident seemingly identified with this projection, given her feeling of ultimate responsibility for Mr. B.) When I came into the room, Mr. B was suddenly inundated with something he had tried to disavow; his split was no longer successful, and he was forced to reconcile the perspective he had worked on with me the previous day, one requiring *joint* responsibility for his improvement. An affront to his projective pressures, this task proved confusing and infuriating despite its potential to generate a kinder introject leading to healthier outcomes. His internal objects were doing battle with this new relationship model. He later requested to be discharged, affirming he would come back to see me in 6 days, which he did.

Mr. B is an example of what Joseph would term the "difficult to reach" patient (Joseph 1975/1989). When an individual introjects an object that is uncaring or hateful, the person may view the self as inherently bad or unworthy of any other form of being treated. Relationships tend to recapitulate this dynamic of loneliness and misattunement, the individual sometimes taking active steps to ensure such outcomes (as Mr. B did by visiting the emergency room). The part of one's mind that *is* capable of growth and affiliative feelings is often hated because it defies the internal object organization seeking to divest the individual of any productive links with others. As a result, patients may *attack* their own ability to join with another in a creative working-through. Thus, moments of connectedness can be quite hard-earned and ephemeral because they can generate anxiety and a need to shut down contact.[6]

While these patients might long to be reached and understood, fostering this link necessitates a gradual (and often painful) working-through. Split-object models may slowly give way to a more "ordinary" object relationship, one endowing self and object with greater nuance and complexity. When such grayness is cultivated, the projected trait of magically and completely taking one's pain away needs to be reassimilated as *one's own* ability to care for oneself, as opposed to viewing such solutions as located exclusively in the outside world. Maintaining the split-object perspective can lead to a repetitive cycle in which one is always seeking concrete solutions to states of distress. Through this lens, Mr. B might have requested a hospital admission because of how difficult it was to locate within his own mind any potential for healing.

---

[6] When thinking about difficulties in making therapeutic contact, one is reminded of Freud's comment that "[n]o stronger impression arises from the resistances during the work of analysis than of there being a force which is defending itself by every possible means against recovery and which is absolutely resolved to hold on to illness and suffering" (Freud 1937/1964, p. 242).

Psychotherapy Settings

Vignette 1

Ms. D was a 22-year-old woman with whom I had been working in psychodynamic therapy for around 6 months at a frequency of three times a week. In recounting her early life, she spoke often of issues surrounding her father, a high-ranking military officer who commonly "barked orders" at the family, as if speaking with his platoon. He was also verbally abusive toward Ms. D and her mother, with the home environment feeling like a "boot camp torture chamber," as she described it. Ms. D was made to feel weak and defective if she showed any "childish emotions," which included laughing, crying, or seeking affection. She idealized her mother and relished the times her father was traveling because they gave her the chance to sleep in the same bed as her mother and "cocoon" with her tightly under the covers. Snuggled together, Ms. D would then ask her mother to hum or sing to her, soothing her to sleep.

She grew up with a fractured sense of who she was and how she was seen by others. She presented to me asking for treatment because she was displeased with the pattern of her romantic relationships. Specifically, she said they tended to oscillate quickly between perfect, Edenic harmony and a nightmarish hell reminiscent of early home life. She told me her boyfriends inevitably became verbally abusive toward her, something she found "familiar and oddly comforting." During the initial stages of a relationship (which never took long to become sexual), she described a feeling of "merger" with her partner. In her words, such a state of oneness would "take me out of this tight, burning skin of mine and allow me to share his. I wouldn't have to think or feel anything on my own anymore. We were one.... Until we weren't; then the skin was ripped open, and nothing made sense anymore."[7]

---

[7] This description is evocative of Esther Bick's (1968) characterization of how external objects can serve the function of a "skin" in holding together parts of one's personality, staving off disintegration anxieties. She stated, "In its most primitive form the parts of the personality are felt to have no binding force amongst themselves and must therefore be held together in a way that is experienced by them passively, by the skin functioning as a boundary. But this internal function of containing the parts of the self is dependent initially on the introjection of an external object, experienced as capable of fulfilling this function.(...) In its absence, the function of projective identification will necessarily continue unabated and all the confusions of identity attending it will be manifest.(...) The need for a containing object would seem, in the infantile unintegrated state, to produce a frantic search for an object—a light, a voice, a smell, or other sensual object—which can hold the attention and thereby be experienced, momentarily at least, as holding the parts of the personality together" (p. 484).

She readily agreed to intensive psychotherapy without questioning the recommendation. She asked to lie on the couch during sessions (as opposed to sitting in the chair), commenting on how soft and welcoming it was. She said, "I may just come here to sleep. You can keep talking, though. It'll be like my mother humming me to sleep." The space I was offering was one to be "crawled into," as though she could nest inside my office and pull the metaphorical covers over both our heads; neither of us would need to think or worry about the nastiness of the outside world. This was a merger fantasy, using the office, the couch, and my words as a covering skin. My speech would serve sensory purposes, massaging her mind to sleep instead of fostering communication and introspection.

This was indeed how I experienced the initial months of treatment. During a typical session, she would bring in a blanket from home, draping herself after removing her shoes and lying back on the couch. Her eyes remained closed or nearly closed for most of the time. In her associations, she spoke mindlessly about her day, emphasizing her grievances about her boyfriend and wondering aloud how to resolve the issues. Anything I said elicited little more than a short silence and a serene countenance of detached bemusement, like a snowflake flitting in front of her eyes and readily evaporating. My words were almost always left in such a state of empty suspension, finding no resonance within her to allow deeper associations to emerge. There was a tedious ease to sessions, and I took for granted the role of soothing, idealized object I was being cast in.

I broke from this role each time I ended a session, something Ms. D found quite jarring. For the first several months, she seemed to experience my saying "we're out of time" as an act of physical violence coming from me. Upon hearing the words, she would freeze, shudder, and open her eyes wide, with a seeming sense of terror taking over. She would slowly gather her belongings, announce loudly when our next appointment was (akin to telling a soldier when to report for duty—"tomorrow, 3 P.M."), and walk out. The pain of the break was mitigated by this imaginary line extending from the 51st minute of one session to the next time we were scheduled to meet, dampening the reality of our separate, individual minds.

One day, Ms. D showed up at my open door 5 minutes before we were scheduled to meet. She looked frazzled and quite displeased.

P: I'm here.
T: I need a couple of minutes.
P: I want to come in now, please. Can't I come in and sit down while you do what you need to?
T: I should probably come get you in a bit.
P: Can I just stand here, then?
T: Let me come get you. (I feel a tightening, burning feeling in my head.)

    P: Are you fucking *serious*? (She turns and walks away.)

I felt tremendous pressure when seeing her at the door, asking to start early. At that threshold, I was being pushed into the role of an object that did not impose limits, did not force her to care for herself at all, and kept her from feeling frustration. The very words I used reflected these pressures—for instance, telling her I needed "a couple" of minutes even though the wait would really be longer and that I should "probably" come get her, implicitly questioning the validity of my own frame. With my choice of language, I was narrowing the gap between us and trying to keep her from feeling too deprived. I waited the 5 minutes and went to retrieve her from the waiting room, expecting a most unpleasant session.

She stomped loudly into the office. It was raining that day, and I noticed her shoes and socks were soaking wet. Ordinarily, she would have taken off her shoes (and maybe even her socks). However, there was nothing ordinary about this session. She kept her shoes on and tossed her blanket into the chair, as opposed to draping it over herself. She sat on the couch instead of lying down. She seemed to be ensuring that the comforts she typically experienced during our sessions were nowhere to be found. I had become a hostile figure, and the environment I offered her needed to be actively shaped into enemy territory.

    P: I'm so fucking mad at you. Asshole, shithead shrink....Making me wait.
        Do you want me to hate you for some reason?
    T: It feels terrible that I made you wait until it was time for our session.
    P: I was like 1 minute early! Two! Whatever! I show up on time, just to get
        turned away.
    T: You felt rejected.
    P: Why can't I sit down while you finish what you're doing?...I was already
        mad at you before I came in here....Yesterday, I was in the middle of
        something important, and you suddenly ended it. I needed more time.
    T: You let me know it wasn't enough time by coming early today. It feels as
        if I keep hurting you by turning you away.
    (Silence)
    P: I can't breathe....(She starts crying.) It's like my skin is burning off of me.
        I want to scream at everything. I woke up, thinking "I have to go see
        that stupid shithead shrink."
    T: That stupid shithead shrink...
    P: It was going away, then you turned me away, and it came back.

My anxiety levels were rising steadily, especially since she was staring intently into my eyes during this exchange and delivering her choice adjectives about me with a scathing, growling inflection. I had trouble thinking and at several moments wondered if I should just tell her to come back the next day, feeling no productive work could be done in the current climate. However, I knew something very powerful was being lived between us and required attention. This was a vertiginous departure from the comforts of "good object land," a place where I was held in much higher esteem. The aggressive dimensions of her internal object world had been split off and kept outside the protective boundary of the tight covers. By asserting the frame, I denied her a sense of merger, tearing open the "second skin" (Bick 1968) and confronting us with the aspects of her psyche we had colluded in ignoring thus far.

Crucially, I felt Ms. D was hopeful that her distress could be talked about and processed. After all, despite her frustration with me, she had chosen to come in. When forced to wait after arriving early, she did not leave but waited for us to start on time. As tense and uncomfortable as our encounter was, it is endlessly preferable for patients to come to sessions and tell me they hate me as opposed to acting out their hatred by not showing up.

This is not to suggest that such violent emotions are easy to metabolize. I was struggling immensely with the sharp words she was throwing at me, as evidenced by how I could only echo them back to her (in my last intervention). This was my way of suspending them between us until I could find a way to detoxify them and make them "thinkable." I was admittedly overwhelmed and in something of a daze. My situation was one that Ms. D had likely lived through many times during childhood. She had often been berated by her terrifying father, with no protective or containing object available to help her make sense of the experience. She was left feeling dazed and confused, desperately trying to assimilate something she did not have the ability to comprehend. The session continued.

> T: Maybe… (She cuts in.)
> P: Maybe *what*? (She sounds *very* angry.)
> T: You're not giving yourself much space to breathe in here either.…Neither of us can fully express ourselves.
> P: It's like with my father (*angrily*). Any time I had something to ask him, he'd just unleash his "What do you want *now*?"
> T: There was only space for one person at a time. One person would be shouting and the other would be unable to think or even breathe.

As Ms. D was faced with the hostile, rejecting object I quickly became, we recapitulated an early scene in which her powerlessness was terribly exposed. She could either submit or attempt to adopt an active role in the object relationship, claiming a sense of dominance and control. When at the mercy of a terrifying figure, one mode of adaptation is through "identification with the aggressor" (Ferenczi 1949), grafting onto oneself the habits and postures of the feared object. By turning passive into active in such a way, the mind of the aggressor becomes "knowable" and less threatening. Ms. D's choice to remain in her "gear," no matter how spotted and wet, perhaps suggested she was coming back into my office in "battle mode," adopting the militaristic stance of an intolerant object. I tried to keep my thinking afloat and complete that hanging "maybe" that had been uprooted.

> T: I was saying maybe it [the feeling of anger and rejection] needed to come back so we could work on it together.

She remained silent for 30 seconds and started rocking back and forth, appearing perplexed about how to take my response. As mentioned in Chapter 6, a mind that retains its thinking capacities while being bombarded with projections may be infuriating to the projector.[8] I felt the escalating intensity of her statements was a desperate attempt to communicate just *how* potentially disintegrating the emotions she was dealing with really were. She likely noticed my shaky voice and rigid posture, which reached a peak just as her affect did....Although I worried that our relationship might crumble under the pressure, I knew there was some part within her, *somewhere*, that kept her coming back and that wanted our work to continue. I tried hard to remain in contact with that part of her despite contrary pressures.

> (The patient stops rocking and breaks the silence.)
> P: Together....How could you ever get me?...How do we heal this? In *real* life, if I behaved like this with my boyfriend, I'd have gotten my ass beaten and been told to fuck off.
> T: Perhaps what we went through was the only way of understanding something that had been trying to find its way into our work, something we may have been ignoring all this time. Since it didn't destroy us, we can welcome it and try to learn from it.
> P: Hmm. Fine. Welcome, you monster! I'm kidding. (She smiles.)
> T: It probably feels better to kid about a monster than to fear one.
> P: But...I don't know how else *to* behave with people. I never knew any in between....Will this destroy everything we've done so far? Once I'm in "that place" with someone, I feel like that's the end. Time to move on, find some new angel, and wait for *that* to turn, too.
> T: You feel our entire relationship needs to be defined by its lowest point. This keeps us stuck in a damaged place, unable to grow or heal; it also keeps us from seeing our time together as an evolving narrative, a progression with some high points and some low ones.
> P: (Ponders what I said.) I never looked at it that way....Maybe you *aren't* stuck in a place where you always have to hate me—or me you—because of today. I guess what my dad showed me was that when something

---

[8] To reference Bion (1959), "Should the breast be felt as fundamentally understanding, it has been transformed by the infant's envy and hate into an object whose devouring greed has as its aim the introjection of the infant's projective identifications in order to destroy them. This can show in the patient's belief that the analyst strives, by understanding the patient, to drive him insane" (p. 314).

bad happens, you hold a grudge forever....The bad thing is what *de-fines* the relationship, like a compass guiding how you think, but there is only one direction to follow. He told me, "Never let things go." *I was never forgiven if he thought I did something bad. Even if 10 or 15 years had passed, it would be pulled out of the mental archive, like some horrible hidden file, to remind me that he had some superiority over me....He had this damaged image of me in his mind, and I was never seen as anything beyond that.*

This was a pivotal episode in our treatment. During earlier sessions, the potential for me to become the all-bad object was disavowed, as we (unconsciously) colluded to keep the surface still. However, monsters can lurk beneath calm waters, and it is crucial that we recognize the worries about what might happen if patients expand their thinking of us beyond two-dimensional, split modes. Ms. D could not afford to imagine our relationship being other than what she had with her mother, lest it be dominated by terror and destructiveness. These were the two split-object modes with which she was familiar. When she turned up early and I made her wait, I failed to live up to the idealization, and, suddenly, my potential to be a monstrous, bad object flooded her. Her narrow view of me as all good suddenly shifted to its all-bad counterpart, and I was treated accordingly. As my anxiety and tension escalated in the session, I felt the urge at times to respond to her with hostility—a pull to reenact a damaging object relationship through projective identification. I needed to access my mind beyond these part-object pressures in order to work with her therapeutically.

When the therapeutic dyad is confronted by the violence of split-off aspects of the patient's psyche, there may be tremendous anxiety that this will destroy the therapist and the relationship. (This justifies the need to defend so strongly against allowing these disavowed elements to cloud the patient's perception of us in the first place.) When such destruction does *not* occur, we are showing we are sturdy enough to access and work through something that seemed unbearable and terrifying for patients.[9] Through this process, patients can reassimilate what was split off as something of their own, contributing to a greater sense of wholeness and to a dimensionality that may have been denied to them earlier (as in the case of Ms. D).

---

[9] As Winnicott (1969) noted, the subject comes to appreciate the object's ability to survive the self's aggressiveness. In "The Use of an Object," he imagined the following exchange: "The subject says to the object: 'I destroyed you,' and the object is there to receive the communication. From now on the subject says: 'Hullo object!' 'I destroyed you.' 'I love you.' 'You have value for me because of your survival of my destruction of you'" (p. 713).

For this to happen, we must create space for the bad object to become manifest because it may have much to teach us about the patient's internal world. As Charles and colleagues (2019) stated, "[R]elational strivings underlie even the most threatening of behaviors" (p. 89), a concept that can help us keep the potential for connectedness and healing in mind in the midst of a transference storm.

PSYCHIC IMMOBILITY, OMNISCIENCE, AND ATTACKS ON THINKING

The last vignette illustrated how some therapeutic wiggle room can be found amid pressures to conform to part-object roles. However, this is not always the case. At times, patients may feel they can only hold themselves together by avoiding *any* change to their current psychic construct; it is like a completed jigsaw puzzle that cannot have a single piece removed, lest the integrity of the image be compromised. In such instances, "psychic change is experienced as catastrophic, since the changes disintegrate the sense of self-continuity. When this happens the subjective experience is one of fragmentation. In these circumstances, in order to preserve a sense of continuity of existence, *all* change must be resisted and no new experience allowed to emerge" (Britton 1992, p.112; emphasis in original).

Patients might not allow us to become anything *other* than what their projections dictate. After all, part-object relationships are antidotes to the perils of uncertainty. For patients operating in a paranoid-schizoid mode, *any* movement can feel like stepping onto a minefield. Paralysis is safer than risking destruction. A patient of mine would become very anxious whenever I offered a perspective he had not considered; after I spoke, he would curl up into a ball on the couch, rocking side to side while repeating, "I'm okay, I'm okay, I'm okay." He was using words to insulate himself from me and my destabilizing mind.

The potential for growth can be sacrificed to ensure sameness. There are sessions in which I receive the very clear message that no matter *what* I have to say, it is unwelcome. The very fact that I am speaking *at all* is an affront to the need for stillness. I had a patient who would jump in as soon as I started talking, rolling his eyes, correcting my grammar, or accusing me of being a "fortune cookie therapist." I was denied access to his mind at every turn, lest I say something to disturb its tenuous sense of equilibrium.

Sameness can also be enforced by adopting an omniscient approach to life's complexities. In sessions, patients might try to convince us that they "have everything figured out" regarding their conflicts and emotions. Some patients might even come to therapy to *prove* there is nothing more to be learned and that our help is not needed. For instance, this may occur if the person coming to treatment is doing so at the behest of a third party (e.g., spouse, employer, friend), someone the patient is committed to proving wrong. Thus, we can be rendered useless before being given the chance to develop our own thoughts about what is happening with the patient. This dynamic accords with the defensive structure outlined—we are not *supposed* to think but rather agree with the patient's conception of reality and jettison any alternative perspectives our minds might afford. Under pressure, we might end up agreeing with patients—"Yes, this is just a chemical imbalance. You have good insight into your childhood and what contributed to your problems. There is no need to do any talk therapy." Indeed, at such junctures, we might try to implement some *other* way of conducting therapy, dropping the open, exploratory stance. We may look for ways to make ourselves *needed* by these patients, grasping for something we can give them that they cannot provide for themselves. Strategies include offering concrete advice on outside matters, self-disclosing indiscriminately (drawing the patient's interest to the content of our minds and lives), or even prescribing medications when there is no compelling clinical indication. Although there might be the urge to override a patient's attempts to devalue us, we should endeavor to regain therapeutic footing, keeping in mind that our feelings of impotence and uselessness may be vividly illustrating the patient's internal object world.

Use of omniscience can be observed in the "thick-skinned" narcissistic patient (Rosenfeld 1987), whose fragile ego demands a hypertrophied, grandiose conception of self, accompanied by a need to devalue the intelligence and importance of others.[10] People exist as part-object extensions to be kept in awe of this individual's talents and intellect. No one can be allowed to offer insights that have not already been thought of by this individual, given the threat this poses to self-sufficiency and omniscience. Lest the prowess of other minds generate envy, they need to be attacked and ridiculed.[11] This is problematic in therapy, of course, because a therapist needs to be kept in check as

---

[10] Rosenfeld (1987) contrasted this with "thin-skinned" narcissistic patients, who were "hypersensitive and easily hurt in everyday life (…) In my experience the 'thin-skinned' narcissistic patients were, as children, repeatedly severely traumatized in their feelings of self-regard. They seem to have felt persistently and excessively inferior, ashamed and vulnerable, and rejected by everybody" (p. 274). Conceptually, there are similarities between thin-skinned narcissism and the injurious impact of early empathic failures, as described by Heinz Kohut. This perspective informs the technical approach of some self psychology therapists, who often focus on providing an empathic "selfobject" presence for patients to help redress these early environmental deficits.

[11] This can factor into romantic relationships as well. Otto Kernberg (2011) suggested that narcissistic patients "have great difficulty in maintaining a stable love relation. The unconscious envy of the sexual partner, defended against by a process of relentless devaluation is a dominant dynamic of these cases" (p. 1502).

the patient maintains a closed-circuit loop of associations that leaves no space for additional insights. Somehow the patient is sufferer and healer all in one; the therapist becomes a mere observer, an audience member to a one-person play with no room in the script for additional characters. Through exclusion and devaluing, patients with thick-skinned narcissism are heavily defended against exposing their unstable and fragile ego structures (Kernberg 1967). In sessions, if the therapist tries to be helpful or collaborative (as opposed to simply basking in the patient's brilliance), this can be experienced as a shaming indictment of the patient's ineptitude and lack of insight. Envy and resentment may dominate, with a doubling down of efforts to erase the significance and value of the therapist's contributions. In some cases, treatment is abandoned entirely, "proving" beyond doubt that the therapist is disposable.

This section outlined how the ability to think can become undone, both in self and object. I will now present a vignette to illustrate how some of these dynamics manifest in treatment.

Vignette 2

Prior to my 3-week vacation, Mr. J (a man who had experienced significant childhood neglect and with whom I had been working for some years) made the following statement:

> P: Look, I'm going to ask you this, and I don't want you to do your usual thing of "discussing it." I want you to take a couple more weeks off from meeting with me, and we can meet in like 6 weeks.

I was puzzled by this "request"—which he posed almost as a demand—and by how resistant he was to exploring the meaning of his comment (he was usually quite introspective and self-aware). The session proceeded:

> T: You don't want to discuss it.
> P: No, I don't want to make a big deal of it. There's no meaning behind it.
> T: But it seems so important for us to understand this. I'll be available in 4 weeks....
> (Mr. J rolls his eyes and lets out a disgusted sigh. He shifts in his chair, uncrossing and recrossing his legs.)
> P: Look, this is exactly what I *don't* want you to do. *Stop* thinking about it. It's done! You *need* time off from me.
> T: Maybe it feels like I'm taking vacation *because* of how challenging it is to treat you. You may worry that if I don't have enough time off, I won't want to keep working with you when I return.
> P: Yes, exactly. Take more time. I'll be okay.
> T: You seem very concerned about the effect you're having on me. Perhaps you're worried that if we even *try* to look at this together, I'll end up realizing I really *am* tired of working with you and that *no* amount of time off could repair that. (He looks at the floor, seeming more anx-

ious.) Maybe that's why you're pushing me to act without even thinking about it more.
P: I'm not doing this....Please stop....I won't discuss this.

As this discussion went on, I was feeling increasingly flustered, sensing my
empathy slowly draining away. There really *was* the temptation to just throw
my arms up and say, "Fine, you don't want to meet for 2 more weeks? Then
that's what we'll do." But I did try to keep my footing as I considered what
our interaction could teach us about his internal objects.

Given his history, Mr. J knew what it was like to be left behind by those
closest to him. A deepening of our relationship invited the terrifying prospect of these abandoning dynamics being repeated, especially as I became acquainted with his more objectionable features (which he may have associated
with the object's wish to leave him). As he felt more vulnerable and intimate
with me, the hope of being treated differently would spar with his ingrained
template of rejection, one predicated on a noncurious, closed-off, and hateful
object that only tolerated him up to a certain point. The fact that I was taking
any time off (which he instinctively associated with his own negative effects on
me) suggested I could easily become this rejecting object. When Mr. J was faced
with separation, I became the early object that did not care about him in any
sustaining way, dropping him at my convenience without further thought.
If I were to identify as this object, I would need to get away from him for as
long as possible without giving it a second thought (which is exactly what I
was feeling pushed to do). Keeping me from thinking seemed to be the necessary pressure on his end because thinking could only spell catastrophe—
either I would confuse him by not conforming to his projection, or I would
conform *too much* and, by thinking, realize how much I really *did* need to get
away from his badness, which might cause me to leave him forever, as opposed
to being gone for "only" 6 weeks. In the midst of this exchange, I did in fact
notice my brain tightening up and my thinking abilities oozing away. My
thoughts were more concrete and rudimentary; I could tell my mind was at
risk of crumbling altogether.

T: How can I agree to something I don't understand?
P: By doing it.
(Silence for 60 seconds)
T: I'm not playing dumb.... I really want to look at this with you.
P: (Under his breath) You *are* playing dumb....
T: (My annoyance escalates.) Well...I'm available to you in 4 weeks. If you
    want to cancel our next scheduled session, that's up to you.

As my thinking narrowed, my irritation grew, and my responses became
more concrete. Although I knew something powerful was being communi-

cated, I also felt I was not in a state of mind to adequately process it with him. In such a situation, I could only ground myself by reasserting the frame, which I did by *not* agreeing to extend the break. This proved quite useful.

> P: (Pause) *I'm* not going to cancel it....Then *I'm* the jerk....I just don't want to feel dependent on you....It feels like too much sometimes. I don't have other people to talk to. I just want to make sure you're still on board with working with me.

Mr. J's response was striking to me because he made it clear that *I* was the one who needed to take the active role in pushing him away. Through projective identification, I would become the hostile, unthinking, and depriving object he had internalized. When Mr. J was faced with separation (and a possible repetition of the abandoning template), it was harder for him to perceive me as a whole object who could care for him despite being absent. Thus, we needed to endure escalating part-object pressures to shape me into something familiar. As I tried desperately to hold onto my mind and address Mr. J's anxieties, the tension lessened, and we could both begin to think again.

> T: (I feel somewhat more relaxed.) I think, on one level, it would be reassuring if I just went along with your request, since it would align with how you're used to being treated by others and with how you view yourself—as someone people get tired of and need to get away from. But I also think it would be despairing if I were simply to agree to what you proposed, saying, "Oh yes, great idea. See you in 6 weeks." That would confirm that even I, who you've spent so much time working with and trying to find a place of healing with, will inevitably become disgusted with you.
>
> P: (Thinks for around 45 seconds.) Hmm....I hadn't considered that.... Maybe my brain would have gotten to that eventually, but it definitely wasn't something I was thinking when I asked for the break.

In the next chapter, I will transition to discussing the progression from dyadic to triadic forms of relating. During this process, shifts back to paranoid-schizoid modes of functioning may occur when there is difficulty negotiating the depressive position.

KEY POINTS

- The pull toward reenactment, based on projective identification, can become manifest in a number of clinical settings, including in acute care.

- It is important for clinicians to notice the shaping pressures they are under when working with patients, who may have sustained a split-object perspective regarding others that is being relived in the present. This is particularly relevant for patients with a history of traumatic experiences.

- Moments of part-object relating can give way to more genuine, whole-object forms of interaction. This underlines that no matter how challenging a patient might be, we need to remain cognizant of the suffering behind the presentation. It is our job to try to reach the part of the patient's mind that is capable of affiliation and developing more benign ways of relating to self and others.

References

Bick E: The experience of the skin in early object-relations. Int J Psychoanal 49(2):484–486, 1968 5698219

Bion W: Attacks on linking. Int J Psychoanal 40:308–315, 1959

Bollas C: The transformational object. Int J Psychoanal 60(1):97–107, 1979 457346

Britton R: Keeping things in mind. New Library of Psychoanalysis 14:102–113, 1992

Charles M, Dodd Z, Stevens GJ: Aggressive enactments: containing the "no" in clinical work with survivors of abuse. Am J Psychoanal 79(1):69–93, 2019 30760816

Ferenczi S: Confusion of the tongues between the adults and the child—(the language of tenderness and of passion). Int J Psychoanal 30:225–230, 1949

Freud S: Analysis terminable and interminable (1937), in The Standard Edition of the Complete Psychological Works of Sigmund Freud, Vol 23. Translated and edited by Strachey J. London, Hogarth Press, 1964, pp 209–254

Hesse H: The Glass Bead Game (1943). New York, Picador, 2012

Joseph B: The patient who is difficult to reach (1975), in Psychic Equilibrium and Psychic Change: Selected Papers of Betty Joseph. Edited by Feldman M, Spillius EB. New York, Routledge, 1989, pp 75–87

Kernberg O: Borderline personality organization. J Am Psychoanal Assoc 15(3):641–685, 1967 4861171

Kernberg OF: Limitations to the capacity to love. Int J Psychoanal 92(6):1501–1515, 2011 22212039

Miller CWT: Malignant rapprochement and abandonment of the container function in acute psychiatric settings. Free Associations 20B:38–53, 2019

Ogden TH: On projective identification. Int J Psychoanal 60 (Pt 3):357–373, 1979 533737

Rosenfeld H: Afterthought: changing theories and changing techniques in psychoanalysis, in Impasse and Interpretation. Edited by Tuckett D. Hove, East Sussex, UK, Routledge, 1987, pp 265–279

Winnicott DW: The use of an object. Int J Psychoanal 50:711–716, 1969

The Oedipal Situation (Exclusion and Rivalry): Theory

Love has its own dark morality when rivalry enters in.

Thomas Hardy (1895/2016, p. 217)

WHEN I TEACH the psychodynamic dimensions of development to residents, I sometimes pose the question "What is the meaning of life?" Naturally, the responses I receive vary quite widely. I then share my answer, which can be represented as shown in Figure 8–1.

Nothing more to it. The progression from paranoid-schizoid to depressive position is characterized, fundamentally, by a widening in one's perception of the world, moving away from two-person modes of relating, which *always* involve the self, to learning about how people relate *with one another*, beyond those known dyads that include the self. Fundamentally, the Oedipal situation[1] is about dealing with exclusion, with a relationship landscape

---

[1] I have opted for the term *Oedipal situation* as opposed to *Oedipal period*. Just as there is fluctuation between paranoid-schizoid and depressive position functioning, an individual needs to confront and negotiate triangulation throughout life, as will be elucidated further. In effect, Oedipality or triangulation is not a "period" that one traverses once and never faces again but rather a *situation* that inevitably recurs as we are forced to reckon with the endless machinations of nature that are indifferent to our existence. Notably, the term *Oedipus situation* was used by Melanie Klein in her 1928 paper "Early Stages of the Oedipus Conflict" (Klein 1928).

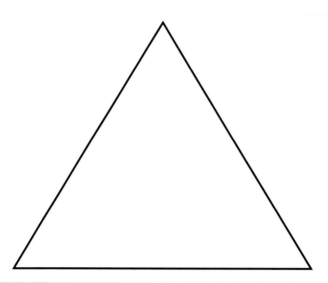

Figure 8–1.   Image of triangulation.

that has disturbingly become triangular. In effect, it is about accommodating a new vertex, one that is *not* directed toward the individual's corner (Figure 8–2).

As the child's awareness of these excluding relationships increases, part-object modes of relating become less viable, a realization that can be quite destabilizing. There is something reassuring about predictability, sameness, and feeling that the world's motions will not outpace our ability to understand them. It can be profoundly unsettling—indeed, despairing—to realize how *little* control we actually have over what takes place around us. As much as we try to project something "knowable" into others, their minds are fundamentally separate and exist beyond our projected understanding of them. What Winnicott thought might be the most difficult task in human development was "the subject's placing of the object outside the area of the subject's omnipotent control, that is, the subject's perception of the object as an external phenomenon, not as a projective entity, in fact recognition of it as an entity in its own right" (Winnicott 1969, p. 713). To accomplish this, we must accept that relationships do not revolve around us, people do not serve functions, the complexity of others extends well beyond our limited understanding of them, and there is a relentlessly forward-moving dimension of reality that does not include or depend on us.

This is not an easy transition to make. After all, in the dyadic, paranoid-schizoid mode of functioning, idealized and persecutory objects dominate the psychic landscape, with little in between. The Oedipal world is one of gray-

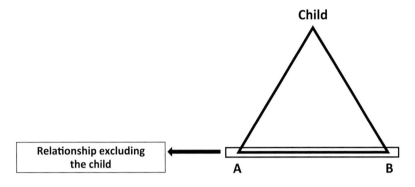

Figure 8-2.   Triangular relationship model, with emphasis on the vertex excluding the child.

ness, and the child is forced to recognize that idealized objects have limitations, demonized objects have positive qualities, and the good and bad traits that were cleanly attributed to split, part-objects are actually different facets of the *same* object. A caregiver who is giving and loving, who picks the child up and playfully swings the latter around, who gives the child ice cream and lets the child stay up late sometimes is the *same* caregiver who needs to attend to the other siblings, who can be testy and tell the child to be quiet, and who sometimes makes the child leave the dinner table *without* dessert when the child does not clean up one's room as told. As the child makes sense of this reality, an increasingly sophisticated perspective emerges, one that recognizes greater nuance in self and others, allowing for whole-object relating to take form.

I will approach the movement from paranoid-schizoid to depressive position as a progression from dyadic to triadic forms of relating. In doing so, I will align depressive position dynamics with the working-through of the Oedipal situation, which deals with rivalry, exclusion, and separateness. Moving toward the depressive position can generate a great deal of pain, anxiety, and grief. Consequently, one might employ "manic defenses" (see "Manic Defenses, Aggression, and Reparation" in this chapter) or revert back to paranoid-schizoid functioning—solutions that are superficially organizing but limiting to healthy psychic development. One does not "move past" the depressive position, nor remain there indefinitely. Rather (as mentioned in Chapter 6, "Developing a Sense of Self: Theory"), a to-and-fro fluctuation between the two positions can be expected over the life span, driven by circumstance and by how one's internal object world is organized. If containing experiences with caregivers have allowed for internalization of a good object, it may be easier to deal with the frustrations of reality, including the need to accept separateness. After all, a more integrated sense of self, predicated on validation and processing of one's internal world by caring figures, will have been fostered, enhancing one's ability to problem solve and self-soothe. For those who did not have these integrating experiences, splitting may persist as a default form of negotiating uncertainty and distress, maintaining a narrowed view of self and object to avoid being invaded by unbearable anxiety. It can be very difficult for such individuals to evolve beyond dyadic forms of relating, with splitting, projective identification, and part-object dynamics dominating their experiences.

In this chapter, I will focus on theoretical aspects of the depressive position and its relation to the Oedipal situation. Given her central role in our understanding of depressive position dynamics, I will be drawing primarily from Melanie Klein's work; however, I will also outline Margaret Mahler's description of the separation-individuation process and contrast it with object relations theory. In the next chapter, I will discuss how fluctuations between paranoid-schizoid and depressive position functioning can present in adult patients in clinical settings. While recognizing there are many different ways of approaching this topic, I have chosen to de-emphasize the sexual focus that often characterizes discussions surrounding the Oedipal situation, because such gendered constructs can feel somewhat anachronistic and not generalizable to contemporary society. Instead, I favor the dimensions of exclusion, rivalry, possession, and grief, aspects more broadly applicable to the human experience and that have significant clinical relevance.[2]

The Depressive Position

The first explicit mentioning of the depressive position was in Klein's paper "A Contribution to the Psychogenesis of Manic Depressive States" (Klein 1935/1975). She elaborated on the concept in future papers, linking it with the Oedipus complex and contrasting it with the earlier, paranoid-schizoid position.[3] She had already, in an earlier paper, reflected on how children's loving gestures toward their objects can serve as reparation attempts after aggressive attacks, suggesting the emergence of guilt (Klein 1927/1975). Indeed, love for the object is represented within the very act of splitting, a defense that keeps all badness away from an all-good object, thus protecting it

---

[2] These aspects have also been the primary emphasis of a number of works within the modern Kleinian literature, further substantiating my approach.

[3] Readers are referred to the following works by Klein for more detail on these concepts: "Mourning and Its Relation to Manic-Depressive States" (Klein 1940/1975), "The Oedipus Complex in the Light of Early Anxieties" (Klein 1945), and "Notes on Some Schizoid Mechanisms" (Klein 1946).

from harm. This is a critical concept when thinking about the progression from paranoid-schizoid to depressive position.[4] In the former, survival of the self is the main consideration. In the latter, there is concern about the state of the external object as well. As detailed earlier, in part-object relating, the child may behave aggressively toward objects felt to be "all bad," infused as they are with the child's own projected destructiveness; these objects are those felt to inflict pain and withhold satisfaction. On the other end of the split are "all-good" objects, felt to be present when the child's needs are satisfied. Over the course of development, the child comes to realize that there are not "good objects" and "bad objects" but rather that an individual object can have *both* good and bad traits. This means coming to terms with the fact that an object viewed as all good may have been treated aggressively at times, when the child was distressed and experiencing this object as a distinct, all-bad one. Awareness of this can be quite painful for the child, who may feel that real damage has been done to cherished objects, resulting in a sense of guilt and a wish to repair.

There is an association between the depressive position and an experience akin to mourning. The split-object constructs of the paranoid-schizoid position, if nothing else, kept matters simple. The child could have a sense of control over the object through projective identification. Crucially, the perspective of the other never needed to be taken into account. Objects could be viewed as containing all the good in the world and thus the providers of nurturance, love, comfort, and safety. On the other end, an all-bad

---

[4] Klein discussed depressive position functioning as emerging quite early in the infant's life (around 4 months of age). As it was not possible to know the subjective experience of a young child, especially in preverbal periods, Klein utilized clinical work and accounts from older children to retroactively attribute reported states of mind to earlier periods. I have found it useful to align triadic or Oedipal-level dynamics with the emergence of the capacity for mentalization (i.e., taking on the perspectives of others); this is a crucial aspect of triangulated relationships, because one can appreciate that others may have opinions and viewpoints different from one's own. This also ushers in the capacity to care about how the other feels, allowing for guilt to be experienced. I have delineated the emergence of these capacities at around the age of 3 years. I am in agreement with Freud's timeline for the Oedipal situation (around 3–5 years of age, aligned with his phallic stage), a period when depressive position dynamics are being negotiated. While recognizing that some of the depressive position struggles may be present before this time (indeed, empathic concern for others has been shown to start within the first year of life and evolve throughout childhood [Davidov et al. 2021; Phillips et al. 2002]), I believe the extant body of neurobiological and child development research suggests the relevant dimensions and tasks of this position will most noticeably take shape around 3 years of age.

object contained all the evil and disgusting bits the child projected into it. It could be abused and attacked for the vile thing it was, the child not needing to worry about how the object was experiencing such viciousness. In the depressive position, all simplifications are given up. *No one* is all good or all bad. The child is not just a helpless victim of the all-bad object's hatefulness. Rather, the child *contains* odious and aggressive traits that need to be somehow reconciled, as does the real possibility that such traits have done damage to one's objects. To make matters worse, the notion of an all-good object also needs to be abandoned. In other words, the existence of an object that cares *entirely* and *exclusively* about the child, never demands too much, and is able to provide inexhaustible love and comfort when around is an illusion. Instead, this object is gray, complicated, separate, and intermittently available, thus eluding any clear-cut and immutable perceptions of it. This can be a devastating realization, as Paradise is being given up. While the child need not deal with the scary, all-bad object anymore,[5] the depressive position also entails giving up the all-good one. Brushing up against depressive position dynamics is potentially miserable—this is suggested by the very term *depressive*. Yet working through this transition, as opposed to defending against it, allows us to appreciate how rich, creative, and exciting the world can be if we view complexity and unpredictability as factors *enabling* growth, as opposed to limiting it. I mention the idea of working through the depressive position because it is indeed a process. Viewing objects as all good or all bad will lessen gradually as caregivers help the developing child make sense of the latter's internal state and of the limits of reality. To the extent that projected aspects of the child's self are taken in and processed by a receptive object, the child can reclaim (re-introject) these elements as parts of the self. This provides the child with a greater sense of wholeness and decreases the need to resort to primitive defenses in response to frustration. It is through cycles of projection and re-introjection that both self and object acquire nuance and wholeness. As Bion stated, "[A] sense of truth is experienced if the view of an object which is hated can be conjoined to a view of the same object when it is loved and the conjunction confirms that the object experienced by different emotions is the same object" (Bion 1967, p. 119).

While this wholeness is needed to foster a greater sense of autonomy and to advance psychic development beyond the two-dimensionality of split-object viewpoints, it is still undeniable that separateness is painful. A child who felt like the most special creature in the world, delighting in the caregiver's

---

[5] I am not referring to cases in which abuse or severe environmental adversity is taking place, a reality that (as mentioned) may foreclose progression through the depressive position, thus preserving all-good and all-bad percepts.

attention to the child's every move and vocalization, becomes increasingly aware that the caregiver does not seem to have the same disposition toward the child. Rather, there is less fascination with what the latter does; to the child's outrage, the caregiver actually seems to enjoy *other* people in the family unit, whether it be a romantic partner or the child's siblings (though, indeed, it can be *anything* that draws attention away from the child). This is terrible. As Spillius and colleagues (2011) noted,

> Before the object is experienced as whole, absence is not experienced as the loss of something valued but rather as the presence of something bad. The losses experienced in the depressive position are not only concrete losses, such as the loss of the breast, but also loss of omnipotence and loss of the phantasy of a blissfully exclusive relation to the ideal breast or mother. (p. 91)

When the threshold is reached between dyadic functioning and the need to accept "thirds" in one's life, a child may employ strong defensive maneuvers to limit awareness of such unpleasant realities. I will elaborate on some of these strategies next.

Regression

One of the "solutions" to this situation is to move backward, attempting to recapture the simplicity of the paranoid-schizoid position, wherein whole-object separateness and concern for others were not acknowledged. The child may "abandon" the skills previously acquired, behaving like an infant to try to re-create dynamics from early life, when the child was treated as someone incapable of self-sufficiency. In such instances, the child might use baby talk despite being able to use words and sentences. The child may insist on being carried by the caregiver as opposed to walking on one's own. If there is a younger sibling, there might be attempts to displace the little rival—for instance, by "repossessing" the stroller or crib that used to be the older child's domain. These are strategies to recapture the all-good caregiver, whose previous existence eliminated the child's need to recognize *any* autonomous or self-soothing capabilities. During such regressive behaviors, if the desired caregiver response is not obtained, the child might escalate by shrieking, throwing objects, making a mess, rendering oneself inconsolable, and strongly trying to infuse into the caregiver a sense of being a horrible, incompetent (indeed, all-bad) object. After all, in split-object modes, if the object does not conform to an idealized construct through those initial strategies, it will become a persecutory and pain-inflicting object for the child, who will treat it accordingly. It is important for the caregiver (as much as possible) to avoid colluding with the child's regressive gestures. Rather, a sensitive yet firm stance can be adopted, empowering children to use their age-appropriate and hard-earned linguistic and motor skills. The caregiver should also refrain from being overly punitive toward the child's temper tantrums and immature acting-out, which likely reflect the painful and confusing steps involved in the individuation process.

Margaret Mahler was a Hungarian physician whose descriptions of the separation-individuation process in children have important corollaries with the paranoid-schizoid and depressive position dynamics being outlined. Mahler's observations detail the child's cognitive and motor progression over the first years of life, characterizing the move from an initial state of merger or symbiosis (dependent on the physical presence of the caregiver), toward developing autonomy and internalizing the *function* of the object (this last achievement occurring during a substage called *libidinal object constancy*), with physical proximity to the caregiver not being as necessary.[6] This progression occurs in tandem with the child's increasingly complex motor skills. While physical maturation can feel empowering (as the child is able to move about more independently), it also confronts the child with the fascinating and terrifying vastness of the world, which must now be navigated while recognizing the separateness of the caregiver. As she pointed out,

> for the junior toddler [...] the world is his oyster. Libidinal cathexis shifts substantially into the service of the rapidly growing autonomous ego and its functions, and the child seems to be intoxicated with his own faculties and with the greatness of his world. (...) At the very height of mastery, toward the end of the practicing period, however, it has already begun to dawn on the junior toddler that the world is *not* his oyster; that he must cope with it more or less 'on his own,' very often as a relatively helpless, small, and separate individual, unable to command relief or assistance merely by feeling the need for them or giving voice to that need. (Mahler 1972, pp. 491, 494; emphasis in original)

Over time, the child's heightened need for caregiver proximity gradually lessens, allowing for an increase in autonomous behaviors while retaining a basic sense of safety. This transition is quite challenging because it places individuation demands on the child, who may feel quite ill prepared to face them. These struggles reach their peak during the substage termed *rapprochement* (from the French for "reconciliation" or "approximation"), which takes place around age 15–24 months. During this substage, the child is in a crisis,

---

[6] Briefly, Mahler's substages (and the respective age ranges at which each occurs) are symbiotic (0–4 months), hatching (4–7 months), practicing (7–15 months), rapprochement (15–24 months), and libidinal object constancy (24–36 months). Although she hypothesized that an "autistic" substage might predate the symbiotic one, this idea was later abandoned.

feeling small and overwhelmed by the complexity of the world and wishing for a return to that early state of symbiotic bliss with the caregiver. However, the child's more advanced cognitive, linguistic, and motor skills will not allow for this regressive move to take place. Continuing with Mahler,

> Verbal communication has now become more and more necessary; gestural coercion on the part of the toddler, or mutual preverbal empathy between mother and child, will no longer suffice to attain the child's goal of satisfaction, of well-being. (...) The junior toddler gradually realizes that his love objects (his parents) are separate individuals with their own individual interests. He must gradually and painfully give up his delusion of his own grandeur, often through dramatic fights with mother, less so it seemed to us, with father. This is a crossroad that we have termed the "rapprochement crisis." (Mahler 1972, p. 495)

This crisis can be characterized by acting-out and regressive behaviors; the child may deploy strategies that at an earlier age succeeded in drawing the caregiver in. When such gestures fail to evoke the desired response, there can be a heightening in affect and an intensification in behavioral output. This protest against the object's separateness is also a desperate expression of powerlessness by the child, who feels unprepared to lose the all-good object yet has no viable way of recapturing it.

During *rapprochement*, Mahler advised caution by the caregiver, lest splitting behaviors be reinforced moving forward. She suggested the parent (the mother, in her paper) be "quietly available" (Mahler 1972, p. 495), reciprocally joining with the child in play and encouraging verbal communication; collusion with behavioral acting-out should be avoided. If well negotiated, this crisis will allow for autonomy to prevail over regressive pulls, a crucial step "on the way to object constancy" (Mahler 1972, p. 488), a progression similar to the child's movement toward whole-object relating.

At the heart of the *rapprochement* crisis is the reality confronting the child that the self and the caregiver(s) are separate objects. It is a watershed space in which the caregiver, by sensitively maintaining boundaries, encourages the child to own one's developmental achievements and explore the exciting possibilities that an autonomous life can afford. Such a stance can facilitate healthy navigation of this phase, expanding the scope and dimensionality of a child's sense of self and others (akin to the development of triangular space, a concept I will return to later in this chapter).

Importantly, the child's ability to reach object constancy may be limited by problematic caregiver responses during the *rapprochement* crisis. For example, this can occur when the caregiver 1) acquiesces to regressive demands, collusively encouraging behaviors that ignore the child's developmental achievements, or 2) responds to acting-out with impatience and hostility, forcefully shutting down the behavior in lieu of empathizing with the child's struggles. In both cases, the caregiver adopts a polarized stance toward the child's behaviors, conforming to part-object configurations (all-good and all-bad, respectively). Thus, a whole object is lacking to help scaffold the child through a healthy resolution of the *rapprochement* crisis. Instead, splitting behaviors in the child may be reinforced.[7]

A parallel can be drawn with patients with borderline personality disorder (who frequently employ splitting). For such patients, the therapist's ability to avoid colluding with split-object pressures can prove integrating because this models a separately functioning whole object that retains its value despite setting limits. Of course, this process takes time and might need to withstand initial amplification of projective efforts by the patient. As splitting lessens, however, patients are better able to remain in touch with their own complexity. (As mentioned before, a splitting of the object is accompanied by a splitting of the self. When the object is treated as whole, the self can be as well.)

Inability to nurture a child's individuation process may derive from the caregiver's *own* part-object needs. Perpetuating the child's infantile role can be a source of narcissistic gratification for some caregivers, who may feel threatened by the child's growing autonomy. In such instances, individuation is discouraged, and when regressive behaviors are displayed (for instance, during *rapprochement*), the caregiver *welcomes* the chance to reestablish a dynamic of dependence. This approach is quite problematic and can impede a progression toward healthy separateness.

Of course, even when individuation is well tolerated and encouraged, the caregiver might need to grieve the loss of the child-as-part-object, as a separate existence is consolidated beyond the caregiver's projections. Mahler posited that "some mothers are not able to accept the child's demanding behavior; others cannot tolerate gradual separation—they cannot face the fact that the child is becoming increasingly independent of and separate from them, and is no longer a part of them" (Mahler 1972, p. 495).

Manic Defenses, Aggression, and Reparation

Another strategy that can be adopted when one is moving toward the depressive position is the use of "manic defenses." Although we may traditionally associate mania with bipolar disorder, the term *manic defenses* refers to defensive strategies seeking to minimize the need for and importance of other

---

[7] Of note, Mahler (1972) stated, "We believe that it is during this rapprochement subphase that the foundation for subsequent relatively stable mental health or borderline pathology is laid" (p. 494).

people, favoring instead an inflated, often unrealistic sense of one's own abilities.

There are similarities between the subjective state in a manic phase of bipolar disorder and the psychic function of manic defenses, though these are not to be conflated (because they are quite distinct clinical phenomena). During bipolar mania, the following may be observed: 1) there is an increase in energy and activity level; 2) the individual feels grandiose, larger than life; in effect, the limitations experienced by "ordinary" humans do not apply, with even the most daring of behaviors being pursued without fear of negative outcomes; and 3) the individual feels entirely self-sufficient; indeed, other people may be considered inferior beings who just get in the way of one's inflated sense of possibility. Of course, individuals who are manic have very limited (often absent) insight into their condition. At times, acute mania can lead to very dangerous behaviors, requiring clinical observation in a locked area (e.g., the emergency department or inpatient unit). The more a manic patient is kept in such a constricted setting, the more unsettled the patient becomes. In effect, by undergoing close monitoring and having it suggested that they need clinical help, manic patients are being confronted with a very harsh reality: the wished-for omnipotence and grandiose self-sufficiency are *not* being confirmed by the world around them. As this belief system is challenged and loses its effectiveness, the individual is faced with what was being defended against in the first place (in many instances, feelings of helplessness, anxiety, and fear). It is common for manic episodes to be followed by depressive episodes, uncovering the depleted, melancholic state that was being so strongly fended off through manic elevation.[8]

In early development, manic defenses can serve similarly self-inflating purposes to stave off feelings of dependence. When faced with the separateness of an important object and the grief resulting from this awareness, a child may elevate one's sense of self to lessen any need for the object. After all, depending on it can lead to frustration, loneliness, and mourning. Also, as mentioned earlier in the chapter, progression toward whole-object relating will confront the child with the damage that may have been done to one's objects. This can result in terrible feelings of guilt for having harmed something valued. One strategy the child can use to soften the impact of

---

[8] This is not to suggest that the manic patient is adopting these beliefs or behaviors consciously or volitionally; bipolar disorder is a primary cycling affective disorder, and an untreated manic phase may last for weeks to months. However, the narrative of a manic individual can bear great resemblance to the manic defenses being addressed in this chapter, underlining how rich and meaningful the subjective worlds of our patients are, even when they are very psychiatrically ill. The human experiences the symptoms, irrespective of the diagnosis the person carries.

these unsettling realizations is to devalue the object, making it unnecessary. A devalued object could not *possibly* be something worth mourning or feeling dependent on. Similarly, if the child *has* done harm to an object, it may be less guilt-inducing to think of the latter as being unimportant and disposable. In tandem with devaluing the object, a child might inflate one's *own* perceived abilities, counterbalancing the object's dispensability with self-sufficiency. Thus, manic defenses are characterized by disparagement of the object, omnipotence, and denial.[9] This is problematic because the child values the object yet is trying to come to terms with how aggressive actions might have affected it. Denying the impact of this aggression can be termed *manic reparation*, the "no big deal" defense wherein one dismisses any actual harm one's anger and hatred might have done to the object. Such instances are disturbingly commonplace in later life. We can think of people who, in a fit of rage, strike a loved one and immediately attempt to "undo" the consequences of their actions. They may say, "Oh, you're fine. I barely touched you" or "I don't see anything; you're making a big deal out of nothing." They may also try to process their aggression through projective pressures: "You can hit me back; then we'll be even" or "You were asking for it; you *made* me do it. *I* didn't want to. Why do you make me hit you?" Through manic reparation, perception of reality is shaped to diminish the impact of one's aggressive acts.[10] Although the mind of the offended object may not concur, such an alternative perspective is ignored. Thus, in these manic forms of reparation, there is a *further* devaluing of the object, because the offending individual will be less invested in understanding the object's experience than in finding a way to disavow the harmful effects of one's own actions. Although reparation is attempted (indicating there is *some* recognition of the object's worth), it is infused with hostility (given the strong pressures to devalue the object). This makes actual contact with the other quite complicated, because the state of the object cannot be fully recognized, and the individual engaging in manic reparation cannot take real ownership for aggressive acts.

Some level of manic defensiveness can be expected at the interface between the paranoid-schizoid and depressive positions, because it can be overwhelming to move into the latter too abruptly. The following conditions might facilitate progression toward and a working-through of the depressive

---

[9] Klein stated, "This *disparagement of the object's importance and the contempt for it* is, I think, a specific characteristic of mania" (Klein 1935/1975, p. 163; emphasis in original).

[10] The reader may liken this to gaslighting—trying to convince another person that what one objectively witnessed did not take place or that there is a different explanation for events that shifts culpability or impairment of judgment onto the one being gaslighted.

position: 1) the child does not experience excessive guilt over one's own aggressive behaviors, 2) important objects have *not* been overly damaged by the child's actions, and 3) the child's gestures of love and reparation will be acknowledged and accepted by caregivers. (Of note, both the second and third components require validation and reassurance from external objects; in other words, for the child's internal object configuration to be updated, continued environmental input is critical.) When these conditions are met, children may feel that they too are "good enough" and, critically, that their loving behaviors are *not* clouded in the caregiver's mind by memories of the children's more hostile moments.[11] As Klein stated,

> Omnipotence decreases as the child gradually gains a greater confidence both in his objects and in his reparative powers. He feels that all steps in development, all new achievements are giving pleasure to the people around him and that in this way he expresses his love, counter-balances or undoes the harm done by his aggressive impulses and makes reparation to his injured loved objects. (Klein 1952/1975, p. 75)

When the child can acknowledge one's own aggressiveness without its leading to excessive guilt, the state of the object can be considered, leading to development of empathy. Loving, reparative efforts by the child will be based on what the object might *actually be feeling*; this is different from manic reparation, which seeks to *diminish recognition* of the object's experience to assuage guilt. This sequence is mirrored in the description by Petot of a progression *within* the depressive position from an earlier "manic depressive" phase to a later "depressive reparative" phase (Petot 1991).

The desire to preserve the object is seen in the child's overt reparative gestures; however, as whole-object relating takes form, there will also be recognition that *granting the object a separate existence is in itself a reparative act*. This separateness allows the object to take care of itself and be a healthier and more loving presence during the times it is interacting with the child. Independence in self and object fosters a relationship that can be much more mutually enriching and creative than one characterized by anxiety, persecution, idealization, or omnipotent control.

The "Fragile Good Object"

In the previous section, I outlined the conditions required for a working-through of the depressive position, underlining the need for reassurance from external objects that the child's aggressive urges have not caused too much

---

[11] As Kernberg (2011) noted, "One's capacity to love should function as a major reassurance of one's value" (p. 1513).

harm. When this does *not* take place, the child might feel responsible for in-flicting irreparable damage on esteemed objects. Thus, the reparative powers of love feel endlessly insufficient compared with the destructive impact of hate, leaving the child with a skewed sense of how the self affects others.

A patient (Mr. W) once mentioned that when he was 4 years old, he so longed for his mother's company that when he viewed his parents sitting together talking, he would clamber onto her lap and push his father in the shoulder, trying to "get him away from Mommy." He was unaware at the time that his father was on the verge of leaving the family, which he did very soon after this early memory. Mr. W was blamed by his mother for the fa-ther's departure; she told Mr. W it was his "naughtiness towards Daddy" and "greediness for Mommy" that broke up the family. This is an instance where fantasy collapses into a horrifying reality. Even though Mr. W's actions were developmentally appropriate, he experienced them as a destructive trans-gression on his part. His objects were permanently damaged because of him. Input from external objects did nothing to dissuade him from this conclu-sion; worse, his mother never forgave him, reinforcing his self-view. The in-ternalized object relationship was one in which Mr. W was capable of doing great harm to others irrespective of his intentions. This template signifi-cantly impacted later interactions. Throughout adolescence and adulthood, he went to extreme lengths never to be perceived as disagreeable or hostile. He was known at work as "the guy who never complains." If a higher-level position became available, he would remove his name from consideration if anyone else was in the running. He was very inhibited in romantic relation-ships, telling his partners they were too good for him and that they should always prioritize their own needs over his. Although frequently cheated on or dumped, he never harbored ill will or resentment toward his partners. In therapy, Mr. W would readily agree with just about everything I said. This oc-curred even when it was clear he had not fully grasped the meaning of my words or if concurring with my statement meant abandoning his previously held opinion on a topic. With time, we came to recognize just how threaten-ing it was for him to express himself in any way that could be perceived as going against my views. He felt it was better to preserve the relationship with me even if it meant surrendering his own perspective. After all, showing his true feelings and needs had led to disaster before.

The good object needed during early life is one that welcomes a child's self-expression in its fullness. This object does not demand pure love or sub-mission but knows a child needs to display aggression and other "less desir-able" traits as part of developmental maturation. A child does not act in hostile ways because of malice but because something needs to be commu-nicated and the tools at the child's disposal are limited. When the caregiver can access and help process these expressions in containing ways, the child does not feel at the mercy of internal unrest or that one's own aggression has done terrible harm to the object. As I have discussed, it is problematic if the experience is different—if the child's distress is *not* contained or if the child *does* feel harm has been done to the object through one's less palatable actions. If the child needs to excessively worry about the object's state, this might limit what can be safely expressed, lest further damage be done and additional guilt be incurred. When fullness of expression is not possible, the model of the good object will be narrower, predicated on its limited capacity to meet the child's gestures without being harmed by them. Experiences with this "fragile good object" may be internalized as an object relationship template, later interactions being marked by constant attentiveness to the condition the object is in, keeping oneself in check to avoid disturbing it too much.[12]

The Oedipal Situation

As mentioned, the child's negotiation of the Oedipal situation will align with a working-through of the depressive position. Indeed, these two processes are dimensionally coterminous in the fostering of triangular space in one's life. In previous sections, I focused on how the child's evolving awareness of object separateness challenges dyadic modes of relating, leading to psychic growth or stagnation, depending on environmental factors. In this section, I will expand upon how the relationship *between the caregivers* is experienced by the child.

The challenge during the Oedipal situation is witnessing yet feeling excluded from loving interactions between important objects. The child might experience jealousy, heightened hatred and/or love, possessiveness, omnipotence, devaluing, and a number of other powerful emotions, all directed toward the same objects.

---

[12] In society at large, treating one another as "fragile good objects" might seem like the norm. There is a need to closely monitor how we speak and behave, making sure our speech and actions are not deemed offensive because we wish to stay on each other's good side. Expressing our feelings openly is dangerous because it risks pushing the object too far and being flooded with guilt. Indeed, in popular and social media, it is common for acts of transgression (whether overt or interpreted) to be summarily and mercilessly attacked by the group. In such instances, it is important that the transgressor not be afforded *any* opportunity to mend the damage done through reparative gestures. The "object" has been damaged beyond all repair, and lifelong penance is required.

Freud's Description of the Oedipus Complex

The Oedipus complex was first mentioned by Freud in a letter to Wilhelm Fliess. He wrote, "One single thought of general value has been revealed to me. I have found, in my own case too, falling in love with the mother and jealousy of the father, and I now regard it as a universal event of early childhood" (Freud 1897/1966, p. 265).

Freud located the Oedipus complex within the phallic stage of psychosexual development, occurring between 3 and 5 years of age. His theory posited that boys in this stage have strong desires to kill the father and take possession of the mother. This generates fear of retaliation and castration by the father. He described the opposite configuration for girls traversing this stage (i.e., they wish to possess the father and kill the mother).

For the Oedipal conflict to be properly negotiated, the "desired parent" maintains boundaries but still allows the child closeness, and the "rival parent" also sets limits but avoids overly punitive or frightening stances toward the child. As a result, the child will learn the limits of what is permitted, extending to both aggressive and loving gestures. (Hopefully, fear of punishment will not overly restrict the child's expressions.) Traversal of this stage consolidates the core of the superego, which (according to Freud) becomes more fully installed during the child's progression toward latency (ages 6–11 years). As the child discovers a world outside the home, interacting with teachers and peers, the superego will serve as a moral compass of what is allowed and what is forbidden. I will return to the concept of the superego at the end of this chapter.

At times, psychoanalytic literature (including some of Freud's writings) can seem reductionistic and outdated by framing concepts around the "model" nuclear family composed of biological parents and their offspring. This overreliance has been rightly criticized, and efforts have been made to update analytic insights based on a broader appreciation of how child rearing takes place in modern society. After all, many caregiving permutations are alive and well in the world, with perfectly healthy outcomes stemming from different family dynamics and caregiving roles (Agnafors et al. 2019; Fomby and Cherlin 2007).[13]

---

[13] Readers are referred to the paper by Barratt (2019) for a creative outline of the different functions or roles caregivers can exercise during the Oedipal period, without gendered restrictions or assumptions.

Kleinian and Object Relations Perspectives on the Oedipus Complex

Over the course of her writings, Klein came to date the emergence of Oedipal conflicts and triangulation with the onset of the depressive position (Klein 1952/1975). However, she believed these struggles began earlier than in Freud's description. Namely, the child first becomes aware of separateness when being weaned from the mother's breast. How separateness is experienced will change over time—during the paranoid-schizoid position, caregiver absence may take the form of an all-bad, part-object. As the child progresses toward triangular thinking, absence is psychically reshaped into a temporary separation from a whole object with both good and bad traits. Importantly, there will be an increasing awareness of other whole objects, including the ones responsible for limiting the mother's availability to the child (e.g., father or maternal partner). As the dyadic relationship is slowly given up, feelings of loss and jealousy may result.

As an aside, there is an important distinction between envy and jealousy. As discussed, envy is essentially dyadic, hatred being directed toward an object in possession of traits that are desired by the envious individual. As a result, the individual may attack or attempt to spoil the object in some way. Jealousy is thought of as a *triadic* or three-person process, as exemplified by the Oedipal situation; while traits or parts of an object are envied, whole objects are typically involved in jealousy. Individuals excluded from triangular relationships may feel a sense of inferiority, shame, guilt, resentment or hatred (toward one or both objects), longing for the desired object, and loss. This last aspect is critical in distinguishing envy from jealousy.[14] What is envied is not necessarily something the individual has ever possessed before. In contrast, the jealous person might feel as though one has lost an object previously in one's possession. Rather than wanting to destroy the object, the jealous one wishes to *regain* it, resenting the individual or situation that took it away. Thus, embedded within jealousy is an inherent concern for the desired object, which is not a prominent feature of envy.

Accepting that whole objects relate to one another in loving ways can be quite trying. The parental couple is wiser, bigger, and more powerful and does not always include the child in its activities. Instead, the couple enjoys spending time alone, *away* from the child, who is left feeling excluded and wondering what the couple is up to. This can be profoundly unnerving for a child, leading to a sense of inferiority, powerlessness, and shame. As the all-good part-object gives way to the grayness of whole objects in one's internal orga-

---

[14] On this topic, readers are referred to the enlightening paper by Spielman (1971).

nization, the demotion is dramatic. The feeling of exclusivity and special-ness the child had with the all-good object is lost; the whole object is more frustrating, has several competing priorities, and is disturbingly different from its earlier, all-good version. Children may realize that the special and wonderful place they were afforded in the caregiver's life can be summarily stripped away, leaving them feeling small and foolish.[15]

So, how is this situation traversed? Per Klein, the child gradually gives up Oedipal ambitions, as resentment and guilt interact with love and repara-tion toward one's objects. Ultimately, there is a wish to preserve the loving couple as a model of a creative joining-together of two whole objects. This can serve as an internalized template for the child's own interpersonal rela-tionships later in life. Klein underlined how the loving feelings children have for their parents allow for a waning of the Oedipal situation because a desire to preserve the external and internal parental objects will be fostered (Klein 1945). To quote Spillius and colleagues (2011),

> It is increasingly realised that the same parent who is the object of oedipal desire in one version is the hated rival in the other. Love and guilt-driven re-parative drives then push the individual increasingly towards allowing the couple to come together and relinquishing his desires to overthrow and pos-sess. The emphasis is again different from Freud's: for Klein, the Oedipus complex is eventually resolved primarily through love, rather than through fear of castration and other forms of punishment. (p. 116)

This concept also has clinical relevance, given the intrinsic potential pa-tients have for *both* love and hate. There is sometimes an overemphasis in psychotherapy on "bringing out the anger" patients might have toward the therapist. However, when patients are appreciative of our investment in their well-being, it is not useful to view this as always being defensive. At times, verbalized gratitude should be accepted at face value (while always observing proper frame and technique). Patients need to know that their affiliative ex-pressions have restorative, healing potential and that their past aggressive statements toward us have not irreparably damaged us. Similarly, children

---

[15] Crying at night has been posited as an unconscious, evolutionarily driven strategy used by children to prevent the conception of "rival" siblings. Such a measure could prove "successful" by 1) physically removing the mother from the room as she comes to attend to the child, thus preventing intercourse, and 2) the mother offering the breast as a form of soothing the child. By prolonging amenorrhea, continued breastfeeding can affect the interbirth interval (i.e., the period between birthing different offspring). Children who are weaned or bottle-fed tend to wake up less during the night. For more on this theory, see the article by Haig (2014).

need to know their aggression has not been overpowering and that their love is still capable of preserving their objects.

In a triadic relationship between two parents and their child, each parent gives the latter a degree of access to oneself, without being overly permissive (which can lead to confusion and overstimulation, given the lack of any guard-rails to keep the child's desires within the bounds of safety) or overly restric-tive (which can lead to shame or guilt and a shutting down of spontaneity). As a result, the child emerges from the Oedipal situation with a more realis-tic sense of one's abilities, feeling freed up to play, explore, and learn while experiencing a reassuring and flexible internal boundedness.

Critically, this will have been achieved because the child's parents worked *together* to provide an environment that was simultaneously loving, nurtur-ing, and boundary setting. Such a collaboration will model how two whole objects can join together and create something greater than the pair. In the process, their separate minds co-construct the meaning of parenting through a give-and-take process that is mutually enriching and that does not com-promise their own individualities. Ultimately, there is a realization that the parents can *better* engage in their individual, dyadic exchanges with the child *because* they are also fostering other relationships, particularly with one an-other. Healthier and more realistic object relationships are internalized as the child moves beyond only seeing value in relationships involving the self. In this progression, the child cultivates a space to cherish, admire, and pre-serve relationships from which the child is excluded. Indeed, doing so can provide a sense of *relief*, as an embeddedness in the greater good and benign continuity of the surrounding world is experienced. (It is perhaps such a re-assurance that allows us to fall asleep at night, trusting the world will still be in one piece when we awake.) Britton states,

> The acknowledgement by the child of the parents' relationship with each other unites his psychic world, limiting it to one world shared with his two parents in which different object relationships can exist. The closure of the oedipal tri-angle by the recognition of the link joining the parents provides a limiting boundary for the internal world. It creates what I call a "triangular space"—i.e., a space bounded by the three persons of the oedipal situation and all their po-tential relationships. It includes, therefore, the possibility of being a partici-pant in a relationship and observed by a third person as well as being an observer of a relationship between two people. (...) The capacity to envisage a benign parental relationship influences the development of a space outside the self capable of being observed and thought about, which provides the basis for a belief in a secure and stable world. (Britton 1989, pp. 86–87)

This triangulation may be modeled by one's parents or caregivers but can take on many different variations because a child might be reared by extended family members, foster parents, adoptive parents, siblings, or other providers. Indeed, a *single* caregiver can also show a remarkable ability to model limit setting and appropriate permissiveness while raising a child;[16] in addition, this caregiver may also creatively and productively engage with "excluding" endeavors and tasks (e.g., employment, academic work, caring for other offspring). We can think of the "excluding third" as anything that limits the child's access to the object. When negotiated sensitively, such engagements can render a similar expansion of triangular space within the child, who comes to value and protect the caregiver's connections with matters outside the dyad. Thus, Oedipal dynamics extend well beyond the nuclear model of two parents and their offspring.

Fundamentally, internal triangular space in the child fosters openness to the unknown, a sense of wonder, and a valuing of knowledge and perspectives that were curtailed by paranoid-schizoid, omnipotent, and manic defenses. Acknowledging the wisdom contained in matters and relationships excluding the self allows for better acceptance of grayness. As one's understanding of the world and of oneself becomes three-dimensional, knowledge is forever incomplete and fueled by the unexpected.

If benign triangulation is *not* modeled, the child might feel that the caregivers constitute a couple marked by 1) aggressive domination of one over the other, 2) joint mockery or derision toward the child, 3) inaccessibility of one caregiver and open access to the other (with confusion of boundaries), or 4) "deadening" of both caregivers (i.e., extreme emotional flatness, apathy, and minimal or absent demonstration of love toward one another or their children).[17] These configurations can leave the child confused as to where *any* sense of order or containment can be found. Instead of triangular space being widened to promote growth and creativity, it is violently shut down, maintaining a psychic paralysis and rigidity characteristic of paranoid-schizoid functioning. This internalized model may be carried forward into subsequent relationships, as well as into the therapy setting, leading to feelings of sterility, boredom, deadness, sadism, or lack of progress in sessions. After all, in the individual's internal world, when two people come together, nothing good can be generated, and all that will result is confusion and despair.[18]

---

[16] This underlines the notion that triangular relationships can take place between two people—the same object will at times be attentive to the child, but at other times it will be drawn to different matters (which represent the triangulating third). As will be discussed in the next chapter, triangulation includes moments when the object "relates" to one's own mind, engaging with one's thinking apparatus and creating links that are inaccessible to the observer.

[17] Cf. Britton's concept of the "Oedipal Illusion" (Britton 1989).

Superego

When one thinks of the superego, several immediate definitions might come to mind (e.g., a moral compass, the counterpoint to the id, or the caregivers' internalized prohibitions). However, a unified understanding of what constitutes the superego has eluded psychoanalytic thinkers. I will present here a very brief outline of the superego, integrating key considerations with the material discussed thus far.

Freud introduced the term "super-ego" (as a component of his "structural model") in his work "The Ego and the Id" (Freud 1923/1961).[19] He theorized that the child will move away from cathecting parental figures and will identify with traits of each, progressing into latency with an internalized representation of them that dictates what is forbidden and what is allowed. The superego was thus termed "the heir to the Oedipus complex" (Freud 1923/1961, p. 48). Freud went on to say of the superego, "It is a memorial of the former weakness and dependence of the ego, and the mature ego remains subject to its domination. As the child was once under a compulsion to obey its parents, so the ego submits to the categorical imperative of its super-ego" (Freud 1923/1961, p. 48).

Klein's conception of the superego varied over her career. Despite initial alignment with Freud's timeline, she eventually placed the superego at a much earlier stage. Klein's superego will be made up of introjects from the parents *from the beginning of life*. It may be very harsh but also contains affiliative and loving traits. She stated, "The superego thus acquires both protective and threatening qualities" (Klein 1958, p. 86).

At this point, readers might wonder, "What is the difference between the superego and a child's internal object world?" This is a valid question and one

---

[18] A Calvin and Hobbes comic strip brilliantly depicted a *lack* of generativity when two forces come together (Watterson 1992, pp. 38–39). Calvin is taking a math test and trying to figure out the solution to the problem $6+5$. In his daydream, he imagines himself as a spaceman hooking into one planet and trying to drive it into the other, one being smaller (planet 5) and the other larger (planet 6). When the two collide, they do not create a larger planet, but rather planet 6 *annihilates* planet 5, reducing it to dust. As a result, he answers that $6+5=6$. This makes perfect sense with regard to this form of viewing object relationships. No good can come from the joining of minds; rather, in part-object relating, one mind annihilates the other through projective pressures. In the end, only the content of *one* mind prevails, the other having no staying contribution of its own.

[19] The structural model divides the psyche into id, ego, and superego. This became the favored construct over his previous topographical model, which divided the mental apparatus into unconscious, preconscious, and conscious systems. The topographical model had been presented in *The Interpretation of Dreams* (Freud 1900/1953).

that has been debated. It is especially confusing to try to tease apart these concepts if we adhere to the following tenets: 1) a child is object-seeking from the start of life (Fairbairn 1944), 2) all-good (protective) and all-bad (persecutory) objects will be psychically represented for the child from birth onward, and 3) these objects undergo a constant process of projection and introjection as the child traverses the paranoid-schizoid and depressive positions. In my view, it is indeed more useful to regard the superego as being made up of one's internal objects, as opposed to constructing it as a separate entity altogether.[20] If we think of one's internal object world as being composed of an admixture of prohibiting, punitive, attacking, shaming, bad objects and of permissive, loving, forgiving, encouraging, good objects, we can understand Klein's notion that from the first moments of life onward, a particular internal object equilibrium will be progressively consolidated, based on what is reinforced through interactions with one's environment. The internalized balance between object types will be carried forward into later life, serving as a moral compass. Notably, life experiences will continue to modify and shape an individual's internal object world over time, updating one's sense of possibility and limitation based on an evolving understanding of reality. In other words, the superego is *not* a stagnant entity.

In the next chapter, I present some applications of depressive position dynamics to clinical settings.

KEY POINTS

- The Oedipal situation involves dealing with rivalry and exclusion, which are fundamental and inescapable dimensions in a child's development.

- Moving from part-object to whole-object modes of relating demands an expansion beyond a split, all-good and all-bad understanding of others. This is potentially very painful, given the need to abandon the illusion of an idealized object and to acknowledge that the self contains aggressive traits that were previously assigned to the all-bad object.

---

[20] This equivalence between superego and internal object world has been supported by Rita Riesenberg Malcolm. In one work, she aligns the development of the superego with the evolution of one's internal objects from birth through childhood. She goes on to say, rather directly, that the "superego *is* the internal objects" (Malcolm 1988, p. 159; emphasis in original).

- When the Oedipal situation is properly negotiated, the child comes to appreciate and value relationships that exclude the self, in tandem with a greater sense of autonomy and individuality that is not as dependent on the physical presence of one's objects.

References

Agnafors S, Bladh M, Svedin CG, Sydsjö G: Mental health in young mothers, single mothers and their children. BMC Psychiatry 19(1):112, 2019 30975129

Barratt BB: Oedipality and oedipal complexes reconsidered: on the incest taboo as key to the universality of the human condition. Int J Psychoanal 100(1):7–31, 2019 33945713

Bion W: Second Thoughts: Selected Papers on Psycho-analysis. London, William Heineman Medical Books, 1967

Britton R: The missing link: parental sexuality in the Oedipus complex, in The Oedipus Complex Today: Clinical Implications. Edited by Britton R, Feldman M, O'Shaughnessy E. London, Karnac, 1989, pp 83–101

Davidov M, Paz Y, Roth-Hanania R, et al: Caring babies: concern for others in distress during infancy. Dev Sci 24(2):e13016, 2021 32649796

Fairbairn WRD: Endopsychic structure considered in terms of object-relationships. Int J Psychoanal 25:70–92, 1944

Fomby P, Cherlin AJ: Family instability and child well-being. Am Sociol Rev 72(2):181–204, 2007 21918579

Freud S: Letter 71: extracts from the Fliess papers (1897), in The Standard Edition of the Complete Psychological Works of Sigmund Freud, Vol 1. Translated and edited by Strachey J. London, Hogarth Press, 1966, pp 263–266

Freud S: The interpretation of dreams (first part) (1900), in The Standard Edition of the Complete Psychological Works of Sigmund Freud, Vol 4. Translated and edited by Strachey J. London, Hogarth Press, 1953, pp ix–627

Freud S: The ego and the id (1923), in The Standard Edition of the Complete Psychological Works of Sigmund Freud, Vol 19. Translated and edited by Strachey J. London, Hogarth Press, 1961, pp 1–66

Haig D: Troubled sleep: night waking, breastfeeding and parent-offspring conflict. Evol Med Public Health 2014(1):32–39, 2014 24610432

Hardy T: Jude the Obscure (1895). Norton Critical Edition. New York, WW Norton, 2016

Kernberg OF: Limitations to the capacity to love. Int J Psychoanal 92(6):1501–1515, 2011 22212039

Klein M: Criminal tendencies in normal children (1927), in Love, Guilt and Reparation and Other Works 1921–1945, Vol 1 (The Writings of Melanie Klein). Edited by Money-Kyrle R. New York, Free Press, 1975, pp 170–185

Klein M: Early stages of the Oedipus conflict. Int J Psychoanal 9:167–180, 1928

Klein M: A contribution to the psychogenesis of manic depressive states (1935), in Love, Guilt and Reparation and Other Works 1921–1945, Vol 1 (The Writings of Melanie Klein). Edited by Money-Kyrle R. New York, Free Press, 1975, pp 262–289

Klein M: Mourning and its relation to manic-depressive states (1940), in Love, Guilt and Reparation and Other Works 1921–1945, Vol 1 (The Writings of Melanie Klein). Edited by Money-Kyrle R. New York, Free Press, 1975, pp 344–369

Klein M: The Oedipus complex in the light of early anxieties. Int J Psychoanal 26:11–33, 1945 21006521

Klein M: Notes on some schizoid mechanisms. Int J Psychoanal 27 (Pt 3–4):99–110, 1946 20261821

Klein M: Some theoretical conclusions regarding the emotional life of the infant (1952), in Envy and Gratitude and Other Works 1946–1963. Edited by Khan M. London, Hogarth Press, 1975, pp 61–93

Klein M: On the development of mental functioning. Int J Psychoanal 39(2–4):84–90, 1958 13574941

Mahler MS: Rapprochement subphase of the separation-individuation process. Psychoanal Q 41(4):487–506, 1972 4634589

Malcolm RR: The constitution and operation of the super ego. Psychoanal Psychother 3:149–159, 1988

Petot J-M: Melanie Klein, Vol 2: The Ego and the Good Object, 1932–1960. Madison, CT, International Universities Press, 1991

Phillips AT, Wellman HM, Spelke ES: Infants' ability to connect gaze and emotional expression to intentional action. Cognition 85(1):53–78, 2002 12086713

Spielman PM: Envy and jealousy: an attempt at clarification. Psychoanal Q 40(1):59–82, 1971 5543114

Spillius EB, Milton J, Garvey P, et al: The New Dictionary of Kleinian Thought. New York, Routledge, 2011

Watterson B: Attack of the Deranged Mutant Killer Monster Snow Goons. Kansas City, MO, Andrews & McMeel, 1992

Winnicott DW: The use of an object. Int J Psychoanal 50:711–716, 1969

The Oedipal Situation (Exclusion and Rivalry): Clinical

[The] metaphysical basis of sexual jealousy [is] the fear that there will not be space enough and time enough for oneself.

Harold Bloom (1998, p. 646)

IN THIS CHAPTER I will illustrate depressive position dynamics through clinical material. I will underline how individuals can employ manic defenses and revert to paranoid-schizoid (PS) functioning to stave off the pain and grief associated with the depressive position (D). As mentioned, we can expect fluctuation between the two positions, represented as PS ↔ D (Bion 1963/2018). This oscillation reflects the dynamic equilibrium maintained between less and more integrated states, respectively, informed by an individual's distress tolerance and concurrent environmental demands.

Negotiating the Depressive Position Over Life

Shifts between these positions continue throughout life.[1] It is very difficult to remain in the depressive position unendingly. Perpetual and unrelenting

---

[1] For an enlightening take on how the reworking of the depressive position in adulthood can influence artistic output, readers are referred to Jaques' paper "Death and the Mid-life Crisis" (Jaques 1965).

161

awareness of separation, loss, and limitation is a status few humans would be willing to endure. Falling in love and adoring one's newborn baby are situations in which imagining separateness from the get-go is hardly conducive to building a romantic relationship or bonding experience. A child *needs* to go through a paranoid-schizoid mode of functioning, confronting the limits imposed by reality gradually and in a manner commensurate with the child's processing abilities. Similarly, the parent or caregiver needs to *join* with the child in a merger experience, *becoming* the part-object that is so necessary for the child to develop a sense of self predicated on a containing environment. In providing such an immersive attunement, the caregiver's more reality-based and evolved cognitive capacities can be temporarily suspended. As discussed in Chapter 6 ("Developing a Sense of Self: Theory"), Winnicott likened such a state of heightened sensitivity to an illness from which the caregiver slowly recovers as the infant matures (Winnicott 1956/1992).

Even outside of caregiving or romantic relationships, we cannot expect ourselves to always be in "depressive mode," maintaining a mature and nuanced perspective about every situation we are in. Rather, there are times we simply do not *want* to think. For instance, after a long day at work, we may wish to come home to our partner, pour a drink, and vent about how unreasonable a coworker or employer was. If the partner is to serve an all-good, part-object role, the response we would likely want is mindless validation of our own position, *not* "independent thinking" or a reply such as "Well, have you ever looked at it from *that* person's perspective? Maybe that person thinks *you're* wrong." Maybe, but that drink might end up across the room. We might cry out, "Hey! Just agree with me! Take my side. I don't want to be confronted with anything other than an echo of my opinion."

We may occasionally fall back on inflexible, two-dimensional thinking to give our minds some respite from the demands of a world that is ceaselessly complex and unpredictable. We might binge-watch a mindless show, confident it will not threaten us with new knowledge. We might listen to the same songs or watch the same reruns over and over, repeating lines out loud and laughing at the same punchlines we have heard dozens of times. We enter into the rhythm of predictability, being soothed by the sensory qualities of these familiar sights and sounds.

Optimally, depressive position functioning will predominate. However, occasional contact with the paranoid-schizoid position is not necessarily pathological and indeed can add a measure of excitement to life.[2] Rather, it is *how* this takes place that is key. Healthier forms of engagement with paranoid-

---

[2] Ogden (1989) stated, "The paranoid-schizoid mode provides a good measure of the immediacy and vitality of lived (concretely symbolized) experience" (p. 137).

schizoid dynamics are those that are less absolute, prolonged, or destructive, allowing one to transition back to a depressive position baseline. When this return does *not* take place, issues might arise. Problematic movement toward paranoid-schizoid functioning may account for episodes of "screw it" impulsivity and recklessness (e.g., gambling too much money, having an affair despite its destructive consequences, quitting a stable job in search of adventure). In other words, one abandons a grounded and "ordinary" existence (which was likely quite hard-earned) to chase the excitement promised by an idealized, inflated, and unrealistic conception of life's possibilities. Although these incursions do not always prove eventful, there are times in which serious damage can be wrought on oneself and/or one's objects.

The case examples in this chapter will mainly highlight the *fluctuations* that take place between the two positions, as opposed to outlining some "ideal" representation of how one might continuously remain in a depressive mode.[3] The mind is in constant flux. As therapists, we accompany its movements in one direction or the other while attempting to comprehend the forces impelling it to do so. Such movements can take place rather quickly in sessions, as patients can feel freed up one moment, deepening their associations, and distressed the very next, shutting down further exploration.[4] This oscillation is contingent on how we—as live objects—are being perceived in the here and now of sessions. When we are experienced as safe and benign objects, patients are better able to access their minds and express whatever comes up. When we are experienced as hostile, envious, or accusatory objects, patients may keep their mental content to themselves, meeting us with silence and suspicion. Critically, patients can alternate between these positions within and across sessions.

Mr. L was a 35-year-old man whose parents were constantly traveling for work during his childhood. They were very loving and caring toward him when they were home, but he had to deal with a lot of grief and loneliness during the several-week trips they often took. (He was cared for by his grandparents during these periods.) He had always worried about "wanting too much" from his objects, lest his display of emotions drive them away. During one session in which I felt we were quite synchronized

---

[3] Use of manic defenses will also be presented in the clinical material. As mentioned in Chapter 8, these defenses are not properly part of the paranoid-schizoid or depressive position. Rather, they are used at the interface between the two, as a way of softening the painful transition toward whole-object relating.

[4] As Steiner (1992) noted, "Such fluctuations can take place over months and years as an analysis develops but can also be seen in the fine grain of a session, as moment-to-moment changes" (p. 48).

and collaborating in deepening his associations, the following exchange happened:

> P: I've never felt this close to someone....I know this is a different relationship or whatever, but this feels like something I've never really known.
> T: You feel close to me.
> P: To you *and* to the process. What happens now?

Here Mr. L voiced uncertainty about what relatedness and intimacy entailed. While acknowledging the closeness he felt toward me, it seemed he also needed to put up guardrails to keep *some* distance between us. This was exemplified by his addition of *"and* to the process"; perhaps there was something unsettling about only feeling close to *me*, urging him to make his commitment more impersonal.

> T: We're developing something that feels so rare, so wished for, and so fragile. You're worried it will be snatched from you.
> P: (Tears up.) I feel terrified. Why do we have to always be struggling on our own in life? I'm so thankful....Yet...What do I really know about you? You may be a horrible person. (Straightens up in the chair. Until then he was hunched over.) Maybe you *don't* know, and you're too scared to *tell me* you don't know. You don't know how to understand my feelings. Pull out your prescription pad. That's what you know how to do.
> T: (I'm tense.) You felt close to me, but that became so dangerous so quickly. I needed to become someone who couldn't *possibly* understand you, right as we were talking about how different and wished for this closeness was.
> P: (Relaxes somewhat.) Yeah, something went off in my head, and I was in full-on retreat. I asked you "What happens now?"—which is the same question I asked my father the night before he went on a 3-week trip.... I've replayed that moment over and over in my head...sometimes it comes to me in dreams. But I never remember what his answer was.

This vignette illustrates the movement from a place of whole-object relatedness (aligned with a depressive position mindset) toward one in which such relatedness needed to be attacked and erased. Although initially welcome, my desire to understand him became invasive and persecutory, given his past experiences with objects that show themselves interested but then rip themselves away when he is at his most dependent. Lest he risk such vulnerability, the object is devalued.

As we notice these movements toward and away from connectedness, we have the opportunity to explore with patients what allowed them to draw closer, what it was like being in a place of relatedness, and what led them to retreat from it. If we can process the underlying anxieties with patients (as in this vignette), we can recover our place as a benign object, facilitating further exploration.

Turning Passive Exclusion Into Active Excluding

As discussed, working through the depressive position and Oedipal situation involves dealing with exclusion and separateness. This can be profoundly painful because we must give up the illusion of omnipotence, recognize our limitations in influencing others, and accept that valued objects have interests that do not involve us.

Triangulation dynamics are not limited to childhood but rather are negotiated throughout life in everyday situations. We are constantly at the interface between feeling included, fostering predictability and acceptance, and being psychically uprooted, forced to assimilate new realities that may deemphasize our importance. As we negotiate such shifting circumstances, we might *generate* situations that reaffirm our sense of belonging, while imposing on someone else the burden of feeling left out. Excluding others can feel very gratifying, a form of "turning passive into active" that helps manage one's own anxieties of being cast aside. Such dynamics are relished during latency and adolescence. This is when secret clubs are formed (with their cryptic codes, passwords, and handshakes), as are cliques that clearly delineate who is "in" and who is "out." Part of the draw of these groupings is that some people, no matter what they do, are simply *not allowed* to be a part of them. (Indeed, outsiders may be openly ridiculed *because* they are excluded.) The very cohesion and identity of the group is predicated on the "othering" of certain individuals who are not felt to share the group's characteristics.

Thus, what an excluding individual was subjected to during the Oedipal situation can be symbolically reenacted and maneuvered in ways that feel empowering. Even within minute, seemingly ordinary interactions, there are triangulation dynamics lending themselves to a satisfying exclusion of the other. If two people are discussing a movie in front of someone who they know has not seen it, they might feel inclined to reference particularly interesting parts of it, with increasing affect, signaling to the excluded other just how *exciting* it is to be in the inner circle. The clueless person feels deficient and small for not having watched this movie that somehow became the key to earning acceptance. The use of smart phones can also conjure triangulating dynamics. It is rather common to be speaking to someone who, suddenly, will pull out a phone and start texting someone else, disengaging completely from the speaker. The texter might become increasingly enraptured by the messaging, laughing heartily and showing the speaker how unimportant the latter has become compared with this mysterious, compelling text exchange. (Educators who give lectures might find this example irritatingly relatable.)

Recasting oneself as an "Oedipal victor" in triangular relationships can take on problematic forms, such as romantic affairs. These liaisons offer a convenient forum for splitting. Someone in a long-standing relationship can view the "old" partner as containing everything that is dissatisfying, un-desirable, and boring in life, while projecting all that is good, exciting, and rejuvenating into the "new" partner, who becomes strongly idealized. In-deed, romantic encounters in affairs are often conducted in whisked-away places (e.g., hotels, garages, and other hidden locales), reflecting their very rootlessness. Fantasies can be lived out, with large amounts of money often being expended to maintain the sparkling surface of the all-good relation-ship. Encounters emphasize excitement, fun, expensive meals, lovey-dovey talk, and sex. Any holistic appreciation of what an actual relationship en-tails—with its good and bad aspects—is jettisoned because it interferes with the fantasy. The one who is idealized and chosen over the established partner indeed *feels* special, having excluded the "weak other" who was not capable of maintaining the interest of the love object. Yet despite the desire to sus-tain the powerful role of Oedipal victor, there is a sense of peril. After all, once the idealization fades, the new partner may be relegated to the excluded ver-tex of the triangle. (Indeed, these situations rarely end well, and often the es-tablished relationship is ultimately chosen over the liaison.)

In group dynamics, there is often minimal room for separate, individual thinking. Depending on the nature of the group process, complete adher-ence to dogmatic, inflexible doctrine might be required for membership.[5] Whoever does not agree with the group is at risk of becoming a scapegoat (Girard 1986), containing all the terrible, projected-out bits that the group refuses to see as part of its identity. One either embraces individuality (at the risk of exclusion) or disowns it for acceptance into a relationship that cham-pions mindlessness.[6] Indeed, splitting seems to be at the core of relations be-

---

[5] In his seminal work "Experiences in Groups," Bion (1961/1989) differentiated be-tween "basic assumptions" groups (in which more primitive dynamics predomi-nate, fostered by splitting and projective mechanisms) and "work" groups (in which whole-object relating occurs, allowing for productive exchanges).

[6] Unsurprisingly, often groups and individuals with the strongest opinions on cer-tain matters seem to know the *least* about them. One is reminded of Sir Humphrey Appleby's quip in *Yes, Minister:* "It is folly to increase your knowledge at the expense of your authority" ("The Right to Know," Season 1, Episode 6). This "omniscience of the minimally informed" can be seen as a rejection of any reality quotient re-quiring that one's perspective be updated or modified. The force of this position reflects how threatening it would be to abandon a rigid, all-encompassing under-standing of reality. It is not about learning but rather about *attacking the learning apparatus*; it could be said that the more we know about something, the less certain we become of our opinions on it, since so many alternative perspectives are possi-ble. Those committed to learning see the contradictions as an opportunity to de-velop an enriched and flexible perspective, as opposed to representing a threat to a fixed viewpoint. Truth is rarely straightforward.

tween large groups, including nations and political parties. Choosing a side means adhering to a part-object mode of thinking—only one group is "in the right"; it knows what it is talking about, and (crucially) it is *untainted* by the views of the other side (the "wrong" group). To be part of a group while retaining depressive position thinking would entail viewing one's own group as *not* being omniscient, feeling it might be misguided in some regards, and (something that can be particularly difficult to accept) recognizing that the other group actually has value and might be *right* about certain topics. (Worse yet, perhaps the other side was treated *unfairly* because of the group's preconceptions and hostility.) Even if an individual within a group holds this perspective, expressing it is problematic, given the risk that doing so poses to one's survival within the collective. After all, group cohesion is often predicated on a dilution of *any* individuality threatening sameness.[7] Being part of a group that excludes others can mean sacrificing one's sense of self in order to retain membership. (This is reminiscent of children abandoning aspects of their own personalities, expressiveness, or awareness to ensure the presence and availability of an unpredictable caregiver.)

The struggle between separateness and attachment is a lifelong one. We are, after all, social animals. For instance, in the Penn Psychotherapy Project, 73 patients (ages ranging from 18 to 55 years) engaged in longitudinal psychoanalytic psychotherapy (mean number of sessions, 44) (Luborsky et al. 1980). In this study, the two wishes most frequently identified for these patients were "to be close" and "to assert myself and be independent."

Psychotherapy Settings

The element that the patient internalizes is this function of seeking meaning, and not an object that knows the meaning.

Avner Bergstein (2009, p. 617)

As mentioned previously, patients are constantly dealing with exclusion in psychotherapy. Therapists do not share details of their personal lives, sessions are infrequent and time-limited, and reminders of "rivals" abound. Regarding this last point, a patient might wonder about the therapist's *other* patients (e.g., whether they are "as messed up as [the patient]" or if they are

---

[7] For the application of object relations theory to larger groups (including on the level of national and ethnic identity), readers are referred to the works by Aviram (2007) and Volkan (2009). These authors provide useful insights into the factors leading to prejudice and discrimination, including how large-scale conflict may result.

more compelling and less taxing on the therapist).[8] Patients are also confronted with the fact that their therapists do not live inside their offices. They are not robots that are turned off at the end of the session and stored until next time. Rather, they are living, breathing, and thinking creatures, relating with patients inside sessions and with a vast unknown world outside of them. Patients see wedding rings, pictures on the wall and desk, a therapist's pregnant abdomen, new trinkets on the shelves (perhaps signifying travel or being given a gift), and many other indicators of an active external life. It could be said that the patient is exposed to that "excluding" vertex of the triangle (see Figure 8–2) at the end of every single session, when the therapist says that time is up and other matters become the priority. In fact, the end of the session could be conceptually summed up as the therapist telling the patient, "Right now, I can pay attention to all aspects of my life except for you." (I say this to underline how aggressive the ending of a session can be for a vulnerable patient, something to which we need to be very sensitive.)

I had a patient, Mr. K, who called me on a weekend. As I did not recognize the number, I let it ring and go to voicemail. No message was left. When I met with Mr. K 2 days later, I found out *he* was the caller. As we discussed what had taken place, he reported: "I had a dream last night. It was the weekend. I was running away from my girlfriend and was tripping through the woods. I fell and hurt myself. Whatever was injured, I was unable to move....The only thing I could think to do in the dream was to take out my cell and call you, which I did. You didn't answer, and I knew you were with your wife." The patient was feeling overwhelmed, running through unfamiliar lands without the protection afforded by a dyadic partner (the girlfriend or myself). In a state of paralysis and pain, he reached out to me to try to rescue our partnership, to no avail. His injury was made worse by reflecting on the outside dyad he "knew" I was a part of. In his dream (and perhaps in reality), he imagined I had ignored him to better enjoy the relationship with my wife. Thus, I would flaunt the excluding, powerful couple to him when he was at his most vulnerable.

The Triad in the Therapy Room

In addition to these "outside world" triangulating pulls, there is one that is always present in the psychotherapeutic encounter—the relationship therapists have with their *own minds* (Britton 1989). This creates an excluding vertex in the room despite the supposedly dyadic nature of the interchange. The unpredictability of the therapist's mind can lead to curiosity, anxiety, and

---

[8] Cf. Britton's description of "the other room" (Britton 1998).

fear in the patient, who might like to be privy to the thoughts brewing across the room. Yet patients can never know for sure, and what they *do* know is acquired in limited ways. Although they may greatly value some of the things we say, the unease of not knowing the fullness of our thoughts can lead to attempts to "enter" our minds to create more predictability and oneness, erasing differences in thought. This can be gleaned from statements such as, "I know what you're thinking," "You must think I'm crazy," or "I know you think I'm a terrible person." Sharing one mind and one perspective (even if it is a cruel one) becomes the fantasized solution to the difficulty in allowing separateness of thought. As Joseph (1983) stated,

> [T]here is a very deeply encroaching type of relating, when the patient unconsciously in phantasy projects his mind into the analyst and knows everything that is going on. (...) [I]n phantasy they live in our minds and therefore can talk about missing and gaps and weekends without having the trouble of experiencing them. We as their analysts have to recognize the omnipotence of omnipotence[.] (p. 297)

Sometimes expressions of how our thinking is not appreciated take less subtle forms. Britton spoke of a patient who, when observing the analyst reflecting to himself in silence, shouted, "Stop that fucking thinking!" (Britton 1989, p. 88). As pressures are placed on us to be moved from a thinking position, we try to maintain our grounding and explore what is taking place in the here and now. This will include noticing with patients their movements between welcoming uncertainty (even if this leads to unpleasant feelings) and needing to shut it down at all costs.

How my patients respond to the "conversations" I have with my own mind in sessions provides me with a useful, experience-near sense of the type of object I am to them in that moment. My own technical approach has helped shed light on this dimension. Over time, I have found myself abandoning the need to find the perfect words before I speak; rather, I join my patients in their struggles to describe an endlessly complex inner experience through words. I will sometimes start talking before my thought is actually formulated, with something as inelegant as "I'm thinking that..." or "What comes to mind for *me* is..." (The ellipses indicate my pausing, my "thinking through" as I am speaking.) How the patient responds to my unfolding presence will provide some insight into how my mind is being perceived at the time. I might not be allowed to finish, or there might be a shaking of the head by the patient before I complete my thought. However, frequently, there is a curious and open stance from the patient, who is awaiting my contribution and respecting that I am in the process of conversing with my own mind. This is triangulation in action. Whether I will be allowed to keep my mental footing or be thrown off balance (both while I am speaking and after I have finished) is an important indicator of how the patient is currently experiencing the presence of those two other objects in the room—my mind and me.

Clinical Vignettes

Vignette 1

Ms. K was a 25-year-old woman seeing me for therapy at a frequency of three times per week. She often spoke of wishing life had "short-circuit solutions" and had engaged in a fast-paced and risky lifestyle during adolescence and early adulthood. She initially pressured me to extend our contact outside of therapy but had not succeeded. She also told me she just needed to be "drugged up," calling me "a high-end drug dealer" and saying, "You're like a panhandler who calls yourself a fundraiser. It's all the same, and you're just as dirty." Such strong statements were counterbalanced by moments of remarkable introspection, which had allowed her to make important changes in her life. Yet the pull toward omnipotence and the exciting immediacy of manic solutions, as destructive or illusory as they might prove, always hovered over us. During one session, the following exchange took place:

> T: There's been a lot of back and forth in your life. How you treat yourself is different now.
>
> P: Very different. I treated myself like shit….I expected the same treatment from you. It's how I *deserve* to be treated. I don't think of myself as a thinker, a *thinking* thinker, if that makes any sense. I think of ways *not* to think. But that's how I get myself into trouble…then I have to pick up the pieces…when I'm *sober enough* to do so.
>
> T: When I suggested therapy to you, it was not what you were used to.
>
> P: *Used* to? I *never* had it, Dr. Miller. You have no idea what I…The world I'm in is not like your thinking palace here. I can't carry you with me.
>
> T: You wish you had more of me than what I can give you in sessions.
>
> P: Right. You ask me to trust my mind. Guys don't usually say that, you know. Sometimes I wonder what you're up to, what you *really* think…if you *stop* thinking about me as soon as our sessions end. Do *I* make a difference in *your* mind, too? I *must* be making you carry a bit of me with you, too. Do I?
>
> T: You're asking if you can make an impact on me by sharing your feelings and your thoughts, as opposed to making an impact on me in ways that feel more natural, the "not thinking" ways people relate.
>
> P: The *only* thing that felt natural was relating to people as sex buddies or even just as friends but ones I could do things with. I can't carry our relationship with me outside of here and make someone else do and say the things you do and say. Your brain only exists here.
>
> T: It's not easy talking to me and then having to leave. You open yourself up and may feel I drop you when I end sessions. You're left to deal with

these difficult thoughts and emotions by yourself, even though I helped you experience them.

P: I'm lost and confused, in between. I don't know what to do with myself. I'm not sure what I'm trying to conquer sometimes, other than myself....I sometimes wonder what's the objective of all this....Not to be sad, depressed, or angry....This is the only space in which there is no judgment, or someone else's agenda butting in. I do sometimes wish this could be more....Know you outside of here....I often think about what you'd say if you were with me in certain situations, when I feel sad, or even when I feel happy....I want to take you places that are special to me. I feel I would get to know them all over again, in such wonderful ways....But you have your own life. I don't know what that *is*, but I need to respect that it exists.

Shortly after this exchange, the session ended. Visibly distressed, she quietly gathered her things and left. Her desire to invest in her psychic growth competed with her usual way of viewing and treating herself. The type of object relationship we were fostering, predicated on a careful and serious appreciation of her inner experience, was both heartening and unsettling. The forward movements she had made in life reflected her ability to find value and dimensionality within herself beyond the constrictions of early templates. However, she felt she could only access the worthwhile parts of her mind when she was in session with me. Thus, the limited frequency of our meetings felt terribly depriving.

The next morning, Ms. K came in and started the session:

P: I read about this new medication on a fashion blog. (She names it.) In the reader comments area, someone randomly said that people can experience "bliss." What a weird thing to write! But that's what I want and need. I need that! Please give *that* to me. Please, please, pleeeaaase?

I was strongly taken aback. It was the complete opposite of the place she was in the day before. I felt her swift movement toward immediate "bliss" was an attempt to repel the grief and sadness the other type of session would have her experience. After the previous session ended, remaining alone in that place of vulnerability proved untenable. Defensive strategies were mounted to turn herself into a different type of patient and me into a different type of provider. Ms. K in effect sought to attack the part of her mind that was capable of introspection, affiliation, and growth because it was the *same* part that had led her to feel exposed and in turmoil the day before. In the process, *I* became a mindless prescriber, a "high-end drug dealer" whose only value was in providing her with a miracle pill. Rather than Ms. K. having to grieve my absence between sessions, I could be replaced with something under her control, accessible on command and containing all the projected goodness

I had to offer. This made my actual person disposable and missing me quite unnecessary.

Her use of manic defenses (omnipotence and denial of dependence) shielded her from the pain of acknowledging need and separateness. As Britton suggested, the movement from whole-object to part-object thinking is a shift from "regarding knowledge as composed of parts which is never complete to believing that part of knowledge is the whole and that it is complete" (Britton 2010, p. 200).

After Ms. K's request, I sat in silence, wondering to myself, "Who *is* this person in front of me, and what has she done with the Ms. K from last night?" I said,

> T: You need to gain distance from the closeness our work is creating. . . . Yesterday you recognized you wanted more from me than just therapy but realized it couldn't happen. There's a fantasy this medication will magically solve everything. And it also gives you some control over what it is I'm doing for you.

This seemed to resonate mildly with Ms. K, but it was quickly jettisoned, and the conversation went back to discussing medications, which ultimately I chose not to prescribe.

Vignette 2

Ms. E was a 30-year-old married woman who I was seeing for weekly therapy. She had a cheerful disposition and mostly used her sessions to discuss anxieties about her marriage because she felt her husband had become increasingly distant over the past few months. He would spend several evenings per week away from home, purportedly on call at his job as a first responder. Yet the number of nights he was away exceeded by far the number of shifts he usually worked. When Ms. E asked him about this discrepancy, he said he was trying to earn extra money to pay for some repairs on the house. She wondered about this, because he was always broke and asking *her* for money. Although Ms. E felt some unease about the situation, she typically dismissed the concern by reassuring herself that she knew her husband "better than he knows himself" and that whatever he told her must be the full story.

One day, she came to the session looking bedraggled, with unkempt hair and a puffy, red face, indicating she had been crying. The day before, she learned that her husband had spent large amounts of money on gambling. A collector had shown up at the house demanding to speak with him, claiming he owed over $15,000. Terribly distraught, she questioned her husband when he came home that evening. He confirmed he had effectively squandered all the money in their savings on gambling and escorts. Ms. E gave me a vivid depiction of her internal experience upon hearing this news:

> I looked at him. As he spoke, I felt as though this solid structure, with a sound foundation, that I had built up in my mind as a representation of our marriage came crashing down....it collapsed. A horrible burning sensation filled the inside of my head. I felt a surge of despair come from a place in my body I didn't even know existed. I moaned for...what felt like forever....I moaned, like some baby animal being ripped away from its mother. My goodness....Grief is soul-shattering.

Her self-view had been fractured. For many years, she had only thought of herself within the context of the couple, as though she solely existed in relation to her husband. She said, "I never considered myself an 'I' but always as part of a 'we.'" Ms. E told me she had never experienced this type of disillusionment, which she equated to processing the death of a loved one. She wondered if she would be able to recover from this, if she needed to file for divorce, and if she could ever "find solid ground" again in her life. My role in this session was one of quiet support. I sat with her as she tried to fathom how someone's mind could operate so differently from what she had envisioned. Ms. E had based her sense of a safely operating world on the soundness of her marriage. When its sturdiness faltered, she was invaded by a flurry of confusing and terrifying feelings, offshoots of the disagreeable aspects of reality she had kept out of awareness by positioning her husband as an all-good object whose mind she fully knew. I told her we would take our time to make sense of this overwhelming and confusing turn of events. She left the session feeling much more grounded. She said I had given her space to "think out loud," to string together words into strange sentences that felt like bizarre, other-worldly truths about lives much different from hers, though she knew they applied to *her life*. She told me she would have to take in the reality of what she was telling me, little by little. I reassured her: "Grief dictates its own course, and we will respect the timeline that your mourning requires."

As we continued to discuss this development in subsequent weeks, she became more hopeful and confident she would survive the ordeal. She even excitedly talked about the possibilities life could offer if she were to be independent: "I married so young. There's so much to be lived and enjoyed beyond what I've known. I've made it so I really only see value in myself if it's reflected by him." The communication between Ms. E and her husband had been minimal since the revelation. Although he expressed some regret over his actions, he told Ms. E it was not *that* big of a deal and that he did not understand why she was "so torn up over it."

During one session, Ms. E greeted me with the same cheerful manner she had displayed before the recent stressor, though not since. She started by saying,

> P: I got this figured out. He has a *gambling* problem! Nothing more to it! I told him about my epiphany, and he seemed relieved by it. He agreed he'd go do some CBT [cognitive-behavioral therapy] or something. Things will be just fine. He just needs to tackle this problem. I'll help him with it…we'll deal with it together. It's *our* problem, really. I mean, *I've* fantasized about going to Monte Carlo with some rich, James Bond type, like an exciting fling or something…so who am I to judge him for what he did? It's not like he had any real feelings for these escorts or like he was really spending money on them or anyone else.

I was paralyzed upon hearing these words. As this airtight explanation was rapidly spoken into reality, I found myself unable to assimilate what she was saying, let alone quietly think about it and generate a response. This dynamic persisted throughout the session. When we were 48 minutes in, she looked at her watch (something she had never done before) and said, "Oh, only a minute left. I think we'll stop. Nothing left to do in a minute. Talk to you next week." She walked out. I was left feeling confused and invaded by elements I had trouble incorporating into my psyche. I felt bereft of my place in the working-through process on which we had so thoughtfully been collaborating for the past several weeks, an effort I had felt very engaged in and had sensed she was as well. As the delicate work of mourning progressed, she began to locate within *herself* those valued qualities she had previously projected into her husband. In doing so, she was discovering her sense of self-worth *outside* the part-object confines of an idealized relationship. Within the depressive position, Steiner outlined a stepwise sequence: When faced with the separateness of an object, an individual goes through an initial substage of "fear of loss of the object," during which the person may *take on aspects of* the object and, in some ways, *become it* to ease the pain of mourning it. If this is worked through, the second substage would be "experience of loss of the object," which is what allows for healthy grieving to occur (Steiner 1992).[9] He stated,

> The situation often presents as a kind of paradox because the mourner has somehow to allow his object to go even though he is convinced that he him-

---

[9] It should be noted that this mourning process does not only apply to the death of an object; rather, it is broadly applicable to circumstances demanding progression toward whole-object relating, which necessitates a painful giving up of earlier part-object models.

self will not survive the loss. The work of mourning involves facing this paradox and the despair associated with it. If it is successfully worked through, it leads to the achievement of separateness between the self and the object because it is through mourning that the projective identification is reversed and *parts of the self previously ascribed to the object are returned to the ego.*[10] In this way the object is viewed more realistically, no longer distorted by projections of the self, and the ego is enriched by re-acquiring the parts of the self which had previously been disowned. (Steiner 1992, pp. 54–55; emphasis added)

However, during the process, the pain of separateness may be too much to bear and the pressures against individuation too great. This can result in an effort to move *away* from the second substage of the depressive position. Ms. E had been making progress toward this second substage but was then drawn to an immediate "solution," one she could adopt without need for further grief or working-through. By "knowing" and identifying with what was on her husband's mind, Ms. E found that her dilemma was resolved. In effect, Ms. E's stance could be summarized as follows: "My husband didn't think of anything different from what *I've* thought. I've wanted to squander our money and do some exotic, expensive flirting, too." By appropriating the action and the thought process for herself, she was not threatened by the pain that his separately functioning mind could inflict. In the end, the predictability of attachment was chosen over the uncertain gains of individuating.

Some of these dynamics will be revisited in the chapter on termination, in which I discuss the mourning process of ending psychotherapy and how this is negotiated by patients and providers.

KEY POINTS

- Individuals can oscillate between paranoid-schizoid and depressive positions over the life span.

- Instances that confront us with exclusion or triangulation can lead us to engage in efforts to lessen the pain and grief associated with separateness.

- The clinical encounter will be marked by moments of whole-object/depressive functioning (with greater relatedness and introspection) and part-object/paranoid-schizoid functioning (with a more two-dimensional sense of self and others). Often there will be movements between these positions within the same session.

---

[10] Here the author cites the book edited by King and Steiner (1990).

References

Aviram RB: Object relations and prejudice: from in-group favoritism to out-group hatred. Int J Appl Psychoanal Stud 4:4–14, 2007

Bergstein A: On boredom: a close encounter with encapsulated parts of the psyche. Int J Psychoanal 90(3):613–631, 2009 19580600

Bion W: Experiences in Groups and Other Papers (1961). Hove, East Sussex, UK, Routledge, 1989

Bion W: Elements of Psychoanalysis (1963). Oxford, UK, Routledge, 2018

Bloom H: Shakespeare: The Invention of the Human. New York, Riverhead Books, 1998

Britton R: The missing link: parental sexuality in the Oedipus complex, in The Oedipus Complex Today: Clinical Implications. Edited by Britton R, Feldman M, O'Shaughnessy E. London, Karnac, 1989, pp 83–101

Britton R: The other room and poetic space, in Belief and Imagination: Explorations in Psychoanalysis. Edited by Spillius EB. Hove, East Sussex, UK, Routledge, 1998, pp 120–127

Britton R: Developmental uncertainty versus paranoid regression. Psychoanal Rev 97(2):195–206, 2010 20406051

Girard R: The Scapegoat. Baltimore, MD, Johns Hopkins University Press, 1986

Jaques E: Death and the mid-life crisis. Int J Psychoanal 46(4):502–514, 1965 5866085

Joseph B: On understanding and not understanding: some technical issues. Int J Psychoanal 64 (Pt 3):291–298, 1983 6618778

King P, Steiner R: The Freud-Klein Controversies, 1941–45. London, Routledge, 1990

Luborsky L, Mintz J, Auerbach A, et al: Predicting the outcome of psychotherapy: findings of the Penn Psychotherapy Project. Arch Gen Psychiatry 37(4):471–481, 1980 7362433

Ogden TH: On the concept of an autistic-contiguous position. Int J Psychoanal 70 (Pt 1):127–140, 1989 2535621

Steiner J: The equilibrium between the paranoid-schizoid and the depressive positions. New Library of Psychoanalysis 14:46–58, 1992

Volkan VD: Large-group identity, international relations and psychoanalysis. International Forum of Psychoanalysis 18:206–213, 2009

Winnicott DW: Primary maternal preoccupation (1956), in Through Pediatrics to Psycho-analysis. Edited by Khan M. New York, Routledge, 1992, pp 300–305

A Neuroscientific Perspective on Object Relations

The unconscious is a biological system before it is anything else. To put it as pithily as possibly—and as accurately—the unconscious is a machine for operating an animal.

Cormac McCarthy (2017)

[For] the psychical field, the biological field does in fact play the part of the underlying bedrock.

Sigmund Freud (1937/1964, p. 252)

IN THIS CHAPTER I will outline the relevance of the neurosciences to object relations theory and, more broadly, to the therapeutic action of psychotherapy. Our ability to outline the neurobiological dimensions of psychiatric illness and treatments has developed considerably over the past few decades. Such advances have furthered our understanding of how medications and psychotherapeutic interventions can effect measurable change in tandem with symptom improvement. Of course, this is still an evolving field, and it will never be possible to perfectly map one's subjective experience through functional imaging, epigenetics, or neuroendocrine markers. Two individuals with the *same* psychiatric diagnosis will have endlessly unique emotional and cognitive makeups. Similarly, investigators may appreciate patterns between symptom constellations and particular changes in biological markers, yet each patient's *individual* narrative will always be necessary to provide context to what is being objectively measured. Importantly, shifts in imaging patterns or endocrine markers can be gauged alongside continued discussions with patients to determine how their symptoms have changed. This generates a mutually enriching dialogue wherein objective measures and subjective reports are integrated, allowing for a more holistically informed clinical assessment.

It is well established that psychotherapy is an intervention that affects biological systems (Miller 2017; Miller et al. 2020). Dualistic viewpoints strictly categorizing the effects of psychopharmacology as "biological" and of psychotherapy as "psychological" are increasingly anachronistic. Just as psychotherapy impacts neurobiology, psychotropic medications can influence an individual's subjective experiences, including cognitive appraisal of self and others, emotional responses to new and familiar situations, and even dream content.[1]

Because this book focuses primarily on object relations theory, I will present a neuroscientific understanding of how working relationship models are consolidated based on early experiences with one's objects. This patterning will be encoded on a neural level, along with the affective valence that marked the interactions (akin to one's internalized object relationships). A healthy environment with attuned caregivers facilitates childhood neural development in such a way as to promote proper modulation of affective responses to stimuli, mentalizing and empathic skills, cognitive flexibility, and the ability to learn from experience. With such a substrate in place, new or potentially unsettling situations are better tolerated and can be increasingly handled through psychic processing—in line with the concept of thought modification (Bion 1962). However, if early adversity and *lack* of caregiver attunement predominate, one's ability to manage stress can be quite limited. The individual may have strong and immediate emotional reactions to stimuli, with a neurohormonal cascade that perpetuates anxiety and fear. Because the circuitry needed to "think through" emotionally charged situations is less developed, the individual may engage in more behaviorally oriented solutions, many of which can be quite dangerous. These individuals may show rigidity in thinking and have difficulty assimilating new information. Thus, efforts to *rid oneself* of uncertainty or discomfort are made, as opposed to processing one's internal state to promote psychic growth. Such a response pattern is aligned with "thought evasion" (Bion 1962).

---

[1] Ostow (2004) commented that dreams "provide important clues for the psychopharmacologist regarding the patient's affective state, which in turn determines the psychopharmacologist's next move in treatment" (p. 83).

Early Nervous System Development

In early life, the environment plays a crucial role in optimal central nervous system (CNS) development. Most of the CNS neurogenesis occurs during a span of little over 2 years, with the majority of telencephalic neurons being generated before birth (Silbereis et al. 2016). Gradual, age-appropriate development of different cortical and subcortical areas is contingent on the infant's receiving attuned caregiver responses (Taylor 1969; Thatcher et al. 1987). The *paced* nature of CNS maturation is important to underline. As altricial animals, humans require continued caregiver involvement for longer periods of time. In addition, maturational timelines will vary for different brain areas and pathways, in accordance with increasing cognitive and motor prowess.[2]

During sensitive periods of neural development,[3] a child's experiences will be encoded to create a map of what to expect from the environment. This must happen early and efficiently, because this representation will be important for later autonomous existence. Once encoded, the effects of environmental input are "locked in" on molecular and neuronal levels. Redirecting these pathways becomes *very* difficult, underlining the pronounced, enduring impact of one's early surround. Such encoding will pattern, for instance, interpersonal relationship templates, which become internalized as working models for how the individual will experience self and others moving forward in life (Knudsen 2004; Nelson and Gabard-Durnam 2020; Nelson et al. 2019). Enriched, safe environments can extend the duration of neuroplasticity,[4] allowing for enhanced learning and cognitive flexibility (Gelfo 2019; Rountree-Harrison et al. 2018). Environmental enrichment, in effect, favors play and safe exploration, without undue impingements skewing allocation of resources toward survival strategies.

Protection received from caregivers serves not only to maintain the infant safe physically but also to prevent premature neuroendocrine activation. The stress a child experiences needs to be kept within manageable limits; otherwise, inappropriate elevations in stress hormones may occur, potentially impacting neural development from an early stage. Under stressful circumstances, the hypothalamic-pituitary-adrenal (HPA) axis will trigger the secretion of cortisol, a hormone produced in the zona fasciculata of the adre-

---

[2] The term *neoteny* denotes the protracted physiological timelines needed to ensure adequate learning from the environment and efficiency as an adult.

[3] In humans, this sensitive period corresponds roughly to the first 6 or 7 years of life, though estimates within the neuroscience literature have varied.

[4] *Neuroplasticity* is defined here as the active capacity of the brain to modify neural networks through growth and reorganization.

nal gland. Negative feedback from circulating cortisol then blocks release of corticotropin-releasing hormone from the hypothalamus, terminating the stress response. Ideally, this cascade will be fine-tuned according to a realistic appraisal of the *actual* threat posed by the stimulus one is encountering. When threat estimation is excessive and inappropriate to the circumstances, the neuroendocrine response can be maladaptive, leading to heightened and prolonged cortisol reactivity (Miller 2021).

Amygdala

One of the areas involved in an individual's more immediate reactions to stimuli is the amygdala (so named because of its almond shape). This limbic structure is embedded deep within the medial temporal area and is involved in attribution of emotional valence to stimuli.[5] It has connections to the HPA axis, influencing release of stress hormones (Sherin and Nemeroff 2011). Given its role in fear conditioning and threat response, the amygdala is increasingly recruited as a child begins to explore the environment, navigating the novelty (and potential danger) of situations. Amygdala–HPA axis connectivity triggers a downstream cortisol secretion commensurate with the degree of amygdala activation. Circulating cortisol binds to glucocorticoid receptors (GRs) on the amygdala, inducing further plastic changes in the latter (Honkaniemi et al. 1992). As the child samples the environment, patterns of threat or safety associated with particular stimuli are reinforced, with dynamic neuroendocrine modulation taking place to physiologically subserve these associations. Critically, areas within the amygdala can mature very early in life, neurally consolidating one's default reactions to stimuli in ways that can be difficult to modify (Chareyron et al. 2012; Payne et al. 2010).

Early caregiving dampens the effects of cortisol release in the infant. In preclinical (i.e., nonhuman animal) models, maternal presence can effectively "turn off" GRs in the amygdala, blocking their activation while the offspring is under closer maternal care. In rodents, the first 10 postnatal days (PNDs) constitute the stress hyporesponsive period (SHP), wherein fear learning is blocked and the attachment system is activated (Debiec and Sul-

---

[5] The "limbic system" structures are so termed because of their location near the medial edge (*limbus* in Latin) of the cerebral cortex. They are involved in emotion regulation, memory, appetitive drives, neuroendocrine modulation, and olfaction. Components include areas in the medial and anterior temporal lobes, cingulate gyri, anterior insula, hippocampal formation, amygdala, hypothalamus, mammillary bodies, and several nuclei in the thalamus. (Note, however, that there have been disagreements in the literature as to exactly which combination of structures constitutes the limbic system.)

livan 2017; Sapolsky and Meaney 1986). This point is crucial because attachment is physiologically "learned" in situations of *low* sensed stress, patterning a feeling of safety when around the caregiver. Although there is no clear human equivalent of the SHP, it has been shown that maternal presence can buffer cortisol reactivity in young children (Gunnar and Donzella 2002), suggesting a similar caregiver function in protecting the child from premature fear learning.[6] After PND 10, rodents begin to explore the environment more actively, in tandem with a *decrease* in the level of maternal caregiving; as a result, these young rodents display an increase in both cortisol release and amygdala activation (Debiec and Sullivan 2017). In humans, the first 12 months of life are critical for attachment learning, with motor skills increasing progressively after this period (Sullivan 2012). As the child's exploration of the environment increases, cues signaling safety and threat will be learned, establishing conditioned responses for when these cues (or similar ones) are encountered in the future. The stronger the emotional reaction to a stimulus, the more efficient the neural encoding in the amygdala (compared with emotionally neutral experiences) (Paré 2003). With early life adversity, the HPA axis may be triggered to release cortisol and activate the amygdala prematurely. If amygdala and HPA axis overactivation persists, a baseline of heightened alertness and fear may result, skewing how the child processes novel stimuli. This biased lens can lead to neutral stimuli being encoded as negative or threatening (Gunnar and Quevedo 2007; McLaughlin et al. 2015; Tottenham et al. 2011).

Insula

The insula is a brain structure located in the depth of the lateral fissure. Through extensive connections, it is involved in a number of cognitive and affective tasks. These include fear and perceptual processing, working memory, and mapping of one's interoceptive state. Regarding this last function, the insula is closely connected to the amygdala, generating visceral reactions to situations, as well as temporally and experientially structuring one's patterns of response (Kurth et al. 2010; Uddin et al. 2014). Such an interoceptive mapping provides a holistic sense of events, attending to bodily experience while monitoring emotional responses (Zaki et al. 2012). Notably, insula activation has been described during emotional states with distinctly "visceral" qualities (e.g., romantic love, hatred, guilt, shame, disgust, and appraisal of

---

[6] Interpersonal modulation of physiological arousal also occurs later in life; for instance, physical contact by a significant other prior to exposure to a stressor can decrease cortisol secretion (Ditzen et al. 2007).

disagreeable stimuli) (Bartels and Zeki 2004; Lane et al. 1997; Phillips et al. 1997; Zeki and Romaya 2008).

Hippocampus

The hippocampus is located in the medial temporal lobe. It is involved in episodic (i.e., autobiographical) memory consolidation, encoding factual and contextual data about lived experiences. Hippocampal development is more protracted than that of the amygdala; recall tends to be quite limited for events taking place during the first 3 years of life (the typical timeline for the infantile amnesia period) (Rubin 2000).

As cognitive awareness and contextual understanding of the environment increase, the developing hippocampus will have an inhibitory effect on the amygdala, lessening affect-driven reactions to stimuli (Tallot et al. 2016). However, if the sense of threat is excessive, amygdala activation may override and inhibit input from the hippocampus; thus, access to contextual data will be limited, potentially resulting in fear-based responses. In other words, there is a *reciprocal* inhibition between amygdala and hippocampus. This is relevant, for instance, in posttraumatic stress disorder (PTSD), a condition in which amygdala hyperactivity and heightened autonomic arousal occur in response to cues reminiscent of the original trauma (Milad et al. 2009). As a result, hippocampal input will be inhibited, favoring an emotion-based response driven by amygdala activity.

Given the different maturational timelines between these two areas, an individual may attribute strong valence to environmental stimuli (because of earlier amygdala plasticity), *without access* to hippocampal input (given its relative immaturity) to provide context and perspective to the situation. Thus, lived experiences can be encoded with a strong emotional salience yet without conscious understanding as to why such feelings are present. This may be internalized as a template, with a similar emotional response being evoked when the individual encounters reminders of these early events. Certain psychiatric conditions (e.g., borderline personality disorder [BPD], anxiety disorders, depressive disorders, trauma- and stressor-related disorders) are associated with increased amygdala activity, with limited input from the hippocampus or other cortical areas (Kamphausen et al. 2013; Lemogne et al. 2010; Lu et al. 2012; Minzenberg et al. 2007; Pitman et al. 2012; Shin and Liberzon 2010; Shin et al. 2004, 2006; Somerville et al. 2004). This can lead to rigid, ruminative, and all-or-none thinking, with difficulty expanding one's views beyond the immediate reaction to a situation. Critically, even when new information is being encoded in the hippocampus, it can suffer distortion because of excessive amygdala activity; such faulty processing has been described in victims of childhood abuse (Teicher et al. 2012; Viamontes and

Beitman 2006a). In effect, consolidation of maladaptive neural pathways and heightened neuroendocrine activation may hinder one's ability to learn from experience, because environmental information will be filtered through a negatively biased lens.

One can draw from these data when developing an outline for a neuroscientific model of object relating. A child's mind internalizes the affective tone of interactions with particular caregivers or individuals through the amygdala-insula-hypothalamus connections, and a memory of the event is encoded in the hippocampus. When situations that are similar to those early encounters arise, the corresponding affective reaction may be triggered, and the individual will behave according to the internalized dynamic (Figure 10–1). For instance, a man who grew up around an angry, berating father may have learned to shut down his own emotional responses as a way of assuaging the object and protecting the self. Given the strong encoding in the amygdala, cues *reminiscent* of early father-child interactions can trigger powerful emotional responses. If the man is conversing with an individual who bears *some* (even if minimal) resemblance to his father, it is biologically more economical not to "waste resources" attempting to tease out whether this new person is actually like his father. Rather, given the dangerous unpredictability of the internal object, it is much safer just to assume he *is* and act accordingly. The man may shut down, lowering his head and not wishing to say anything that could be viewed as even remotely provocative. This "angry father/subdued child" dynamic is an object relationship model that can be encoded on a neurobiological level and carried forward as a template for later life. There are unending object-self configurations that can make up one's internal object world. As mentioned, an individual can assume either side of the object relationship when interacting with others. (Adopting the role of the father, in this case, would be an instance of "turning passive into active" or "identification with the aggressor.")

Prefrontal Cortex

Higher cortical areas develop gradually in tandem with the child's increasingly sophisticated cognitive, linguistic, and interpersonal skills. This last domain will include cultivating an awareness of oneself as part of a larger group. Importantly, as mentalizing abilities develop, the perspectives of others will be increasingly taken into account, expanding beyond egocentric viewpoints.

In this section, I will focus on the functional significance of the prefrontal cortex (PFC) during childhood development. In addition to the crucial role it has in speech acquisition, mentalization, empathy, and executive functioning, the PFC is also involved in modulating emotional and behavioral

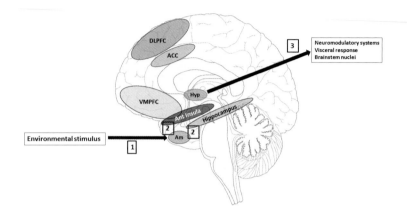

Figure 10–1. Neural cascade in response to stimulus.

Note. The individual is presented with a stimulus, leading to a neural response cascade **(1)**. In addition to thalamic relaying (not depicted), the amygdala is activated, with positive or negative valence being ascribed based on bidirectional amygdala-insula (informing interoceptive awareness) and amygdala-hippocampus (providing contextual data based on episodic memory) connectivity **(2)**. The orbitofrontal cortex (not shown) will also be recruited to gauge reward and risk considerations associated with the stimulus. Informed by this quick process, hypothalamic-pituitary-adrenal axis and brainstem nuclei activation will initiate release of cortisol and monoamine neurotransmitters **(3)**. The degree to which these systems are activated will depend on the level of threat assigned to the stimulus following the described neural processing. (Note that the DLPFC is represented schematically; this is a medial view of the brain, and the DLPFC is situated on the superolateral surface.)

ACC=anterior cingulate cortex; Am=amygdala; Ant Insula=anterior insula; DLPFC = dorsolateral prefrontal cortex; Hyp=hypothalamus; VMPFC=ventromedial prefrontal cortex.

output. In particular, the ventromedial prefrontal cortex (VMPFC) shows increasingly robust connections with the amygdala over the course of development, with notable strengthening starting at preadolescence (Gabard-Durnam et al. 2014). Inhibitory input from the VMPFC onto the amygdala dampens excessive limbic activation when negotiating everyday situations. The VMPFC helps maintain cognitive flexibility, allowing for new information to be assimilated and updating one's evolving understanding of reality (Wang et al. 2017). As will be discussed, the VMPFC is also involved in mentalization and empathic attunement (Amodio and Frith 2006).

When early adversity is excessive, there may be premature, incomplete, and inefficient VMPFC-amygdala coupling (Gee et al. 2013). Because modulation of one's emotional reactions to situations will be limited, the potential increases for affect-driven cognitive appraisals and behaviorally oriented strategies to resolve uncertainty. Instead of accessing the VMPFC when dealing with distress, there may be preferential activation of more dorsal cortical areas (e.g., the dorsolateral prefrontal cortex [DLPFC]). The DLPFC is necessary for executive functioning, but hyperactivity can be associated with cognitive *rigidity*, emotional avoidance, thought evasion, suppression of unwanted memories, and avoidant behaviors toward others. Several psychiatric conditions (e.g., depressive disorders, anxiety disorders, PTSD) are associated with preferential activation of dorsal over ventral cortical areas (Lemogne et al. 2010; Nejad et al. 2013; Pitman et al. 2012; Somerville et al. 2004). This may result in negative, rigid views of self and/or others, cognitions that are commonly described in patients with these disorders.

Limbic and prefrontal cortical activity will determine whether an individual, under given circumstances, will be capable of flexibly integrating information or if emotional arousal will be excessive, leading to greater cognitive rigidity. As Bion pointed out, "An emotional experience that is felt to be painful may initiate an attempt either to evade or to modify the pain according to the capacity of the personality to tolerate frustration" (Bion 1962, p. 48). This is modeled neurobiologically in Figure 10–2.[7]

Containment and Empathy

A child's environment and caregivers are indispensable for adaptive neural development. Early and sustained deprivation can negatively impact brain maturation and contribute to neuropsychiatric disturbances later in life.[8] As mentioned, sufficient caregiver involvement is required in order to avoid premature amygdala plasticity and heightened cortisol reactivity, allowing the child to develop a basic sense of trust and safety. In effect, adaptive neural circuitry can be reinforced and consolidated through experiences of caregiver-child attunement.

Mother-child dyadic interactions activate circuitry involved in positive-negative valence attribution, empathic attunement, and reward. A mother

---

[7] I have described elsewhere how neuroscientific constructs can be applied to Bion's theories on thinking (Miller 2018).

[8] For instance, there is an expansive literature on children who suffered prolonged and severe deprivation in Romanian orphanages during the Ceausescu regime; see, for example, Bos et al. 2011 and Miller 2021. Importantly, some neuropsychiatric sequelae resulting from these experiences have been shown to persist into adolescence and adulthood. Note that for a subset of these children, being adopted into supportive homes slowed or reversed the deleterious impact of earlier deprivation. (However, if adoption occurred after a certain age, adverse effects were not always reversible.)

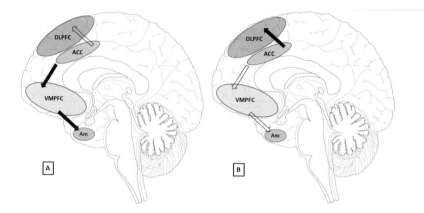

Figure 10–2. Schematic representation of thought modification or
                        evasion.

Note.   The anterior cingulate cortex (ACC) is an area involved in the integration of
emotional responsiveness with higher cortical functions. **(A)** If amygdala (Am) activity is not excessive and one's internal state can be processed, the ACC will route activation toward the ventromedial prefrontal cortex (VMPFC), which dampens amygdala activity through inhibitory input, modulating affect and behavior. (This favored pathway activation is represented by the *full arrows*; recruitment of the dorsolateral prefrontal cortex [DLPFC] will not be as pronounced, as indicated by the *empty arrow*.) **(B)** If amygdala activity is heightened and one's internal state *cannot* be processed, the ACC-DLPFC pathway will be favored (*full arrow*), resulting in rigidity of thinking and attempts to manage emotional arousal through cognitive control. Limbic modulation will be limited because of impaired VMPFC-amygdala coupling (*empty arrows*), potentially leading to emotion-based and behaviorally oriented responses.

who is able to attune to her child experiences bonding as rewarding, as evidenced by maternal release of dopamine in the mesolimbic pathway (a circuit involved in rewarding or pleasurable experiences) (Atzil et al. 2011; Insel 2003). When her infant is showing distress, a mother activates her *own* medial PFC to soothe the child. In doing so, the mother provides the child with an experience akin to *containment*: she is attuned to the child's distress and gives comfort without being overwhelmed by the situation (Laurent et al. 2011), while the child feels the state of internal unrest has been accessed, processed, and relieved by a loving other. Empathic attunement between caregiver and child allows the latter to establish a sense of self in relation to others, gradually acquiring perspective-taking abilities and understanding what it means to "put oneself in the other person's shoes." Receiving empathic responses from others will be important in consolidating the child's *own* empathic or mentalizing capacities toward others. Parent-child synchrony during the first decade of life has been shown to impact development of neural networks subserving empathic responses in the child (Levy et al. 2019).

Early Adversity and Intergenerational Templates

Research findings have validated the significance of caregiver-child attunement. Indeed, studies focusing on moment-to-moment micro-attunements between mother and infant have shown close mirroring between the dyad's facial expressions and body language (Beebe 2000; Beebe et al. 2012). During these synchronized, attuned states, the mother joins the child in making sense of the surrounding world. This co-construction can be profoundly integrating, giving the child a sense of oneness with a benignly present object.

Impact of Dyadic Misattunement

Akin to a "neural signature," there is a very quick (on the order of milliseconds) maternal circuitry activation that occurs when a mother looks at her child, involving limbic and lower cortical areas (Kringelbach et al. 2008; Leppänen and Nelson 2009; Parsons et al. 2013). These include 1) the fusiform gyrus, involved in facial recognition; 2) the amygdala, involved in attribution of positive or negative valence to stimuli, as well as in recognizing emotional states in other people (including through assessment of facial features); 3) the posterior superior temporal sulcus, involved in analyzing biological motion cues to interpret actions, intentions, and psychological dispositions of others; and 4) the orbitofrontal cortex (OFC), an area activated when the mother is gauging risk-reward considerations of particular situations. The OFC has interconnections with the adjacent VMPFC, recruited during the empathic response. Ostensibly, a mother's ability to attune to her child will be informed by the preceding circuitry activation. If she is not overwhelmed when seeing her child, amygdala activity will not be excessive, and the interaction will be experienced as safe and rewarding.

However, this is not always the case. There are instances when interacting with a child generates an overwhelming affective and autonomic response in caregivers, limiting their ability to provide an attuned, containing experience. The aforementioned circuitry may be implicated in such responses: if a mother looks at her child and feels overly distressed, this may be driven by heightened amygdala activation and risk-reward OFC processing signaling there is something threatening or risky about this interaction. One study assessed neural response patterns in secure and dismissing or insecure mothers when interacting with their young children (Strathearn et al. 2009). Securely attached mothers showed *increased* activation in bilateral medial

PFC, OFC, and ventral striatum (an area containing the nucleus accumbens that receives dopaminergic input during rewarding experiences). In contrast, the dismissing or insecure mothers showed *decreased* activation in the ventral striatum, as well as an *increase* in insula and DLPFC activity; for these mothers, interacting with their children was experienced as distressing, with circuitry activation favoring cognitive control over empathic attunement.

Moments of caregiver misattunement can be quite disorganizing for young children because they lack the cognitive apparatus to process what is happening. In the seminal "still face" experiments, Tronick instructed a mother *not* to provide facial feedback to her young child when the two were interacting (Tronick et al. 1979). This was profoundly unsettling for the child, who became increasingly desperate as attempts to regain the mother's attention proved fruitless. As stated by Cavelzani and Tronick (2016),

> [T]he "still-faced mother" is an experimental model of emotional neglect and the denial of intersubjectivity....The infant almost immediately detects the change, and attempts to solicit the mother's attention and engagement. However, when repeated attempts fail, the infant withdraws, loses postural control.... They learn that their actions have no effect and that they must abandon the goals of mutuality. Such infants increasingly focus their coping behaviors on self-regulation in order to control the negative emotions. (p. 600)

The child may shut down, quietly worry, and save energy resources given the unpredictability of the situation. Mother-child micro-attunement research has outlined the maternal response patterns leading to disorganized attachment styles in the child (Beebe 2000; Beebe et al. 2012). Maternal reactions associated with this outcome include 1) showing surprise, smiling, or looking away when the child is distressed; 2) having a closed-off facial expression; 3) showing disgust; and 4) exhibiting behaviors that are frightening to the child.[9] Children may "mirror" the maternal misattunement, showing closed-off body language themselves (e.g., covering their faces, crossing their arms, or looking away from the mother). In effect, lack of attunement results in the child's feeling invaded by uncontainable distress.

Importantly, what is being registered in the child regarding interpersonal relationship templates can be carried forward and repeated in adult life, including with *one's own* offspring. Thus, maladaptive modes of relating can be perpetuated intergenerationally. Adult attachment interviews have shown that parents' attachment styles can predict those of their children (even before the latter have been born) (van IJzendoorn 1995).

---

[9] A mother who shows *herself* to be frightened may also contribute to disorganized responses in the child (Schuengel et al. 1999; van IJzendoorn et al. 1999).

Effects of Childhood Adversity

Environmental factors in early life may reinforce neural activation patterns favoring cognitive rigidity, as opposed to emotional processing through PFC-limbic modulation. In addition to contributing to heightened amygdala and insula activation, early childhood adversity can result in decreased activity in the VMPFC and OFC (De Brito et al. 2013; Tottenham et al. 2011).[10] Also, processing of rewarding stimuli may be impaired, as indicated by decreased activity in the basal ganglia (Dillon et al. 2009). There are striking similarities between the neural activation pattern seen in a child experiencing adversity and the one previously described for the insecure caregiver. In both instances, there is under-recruitment of the VMPFC, limiting one's ability to modulate emotion-based reactions. Just as attachment schemas can be transmitted intergenerationally (Shah et al. 2010; van IJzendoorn 1995), parental maladaptive neurocircuitry templates may also be replicated in their offspring.

As discussed in earlier chapters, factors *inherent to the child* can limit dyadic resolution of distress through empathic attunement. Interacting with a child who has an insecure or disorganized attachment style can elicit a greater affective response *in the caregiver*, who may feel increasingly frustrated as attempts to soothe the child prove unsuccessful. Imaging studies have shown that during crying episodes, children with insecure attachment styles induce amygdala and insula activation in the mother. Also, disorganized attachment behaviors in the child may lead to decreased maternal activation of ventral cortical areas (Laurent and Ablow 2012). The situation becomes one in which the child's internal state cannot be accessed, causing the mother to feel discouraged and even less able to connect.

Inadequate empathic attunement from caregivers may result in offspring under-recruiting their *own* VMPFC during interactions later in life. In effect, if the caregiver(s) did not provide a model of attunement for the child, the latter will have difficulty attuning to others. Children suffering early maltreatment show impaired connectivity patterns in the VMPFC (Puetz et al. 2017), limiting mentalization capacities and the ability to modulate amygdala activity (Fonagy and Target 1997).

Neurobiological Model of Object Relationships

When early adversity takes place, neurotransmitter receptor expression may be configured in order to *maintain the stress response*, as opposed to mitigating

---

[10] Lower OFC activity can limit realistic appraisal of the rewards and risks of a particular situation, ultimately favoring more immediate, emotion-based assessments.

it. For instance, there will be increased amygdala expression of 5-HT$_{2A}$, an excitatory serotonin receptor subtype (Murnane 2019). From an evolutionary standpoint, organismic fitness may be enhanced by heightening awareness toward the environment, particularly after encountering danger cues. To protect the individual from future harm, plastic brain changes can occur to enable a state of alertness, suspicion, and guardedness.[11] These changes may occur early and be hard to modify. In such instances, there is difficulty objectively appraising stimuli, given the increased limbic reactivity and bias toward emotion-based behaviors. This is not simply a matter of intellectually misinterpreting the possible risks of particular situations. Rather, the threat will be experienced cognitively, affectively, and somatically, fueled by the connectivity between insula and amygdala. As mentioned earlier, insula activation occurs when sensing one's interoceptive or bodily state, including during those intuitive "gut feeling" moments when something feels off on a *visceral* level (though putting the sensation into words may be quite difficult). Just as amygdala hyperactivity might cause an individual to read neutral stimuli as menacing, an overly reactive insula may result in "body prediction errors," wherein there is a sense of bodily or visceral distress or unease without any objective environmental danger. (This has been described in patients with depressive and anxiety disorders [Paulus and Stein 2006].)

Thus, an individual who has suffered early abuse might develop a distorting, persecutory lens through which others are perceived and treated as eminently hostile. The potential for traumatizing reenactments to occur is clear, because the person on the other side of this lens may be drawn into destructive dynamics without mediation of thought. This is the essence of projective identification, wherein certain traits (drawing from internalized templates with earlier figures) are attributed to an object in the present, now felt to be *in possession* of such traits. The projector interacts in ways seeking to confirm that the object is indeed a reissuing of the internalized model. If the object is unable to maintain a thinking stance and help process the situation (through use of alpha-function), identification with the projection and a playing out of the early object relationship template may ensue.

---

[11] The reader is referred to the paper by Raihani and Bell (2019) for an evolutionary understanding of paranoia.

Traumatic Acceleration and Behavioral Reenactment

Quick profits made in chaotic times never last.

Ugetsu (Mizoguchi 1953)

As suggested in previous sections, neural changes can occur in response to environmental peril and uncertainty, given the need to maintain a state of heightened alertness. However, these changes may limit further neural plasticity. Stress can damage developing neurons (partly due to elevation of cortisol and of the excitatory neurotransmitter glutamate). When stress is excessive during sensitive periods of neural development, molecular and cellular mechanisms are activated to protect the brain from suffering further injury (a foreseeable consequence of continued exposure to adversity). Once in place, these "brake-like" factors (e.g., myelination and perineuronal nets) are very difficult to remove. This "developmental acceleration" reflects the environmental demand for resource allocation toward self-preservation and away from gradual physiological maturation. Critically, the reverberations of stress extend beyond neurobiology, impacting behavioral, endocrine, and reproductive dimensions as well. There is an approximation between stress-induced biobehavioral changes and psychoanalytic descriptions of the impact of early abuse. In *Female Sexuality* (1931), Freud wrote that real instances of seduction may accelerate Oedipal development in young girls; he stated, "The effect of seduction has long been familiar to us and [...] may hasten the child's sexual development and bring it to maturity" (Freud 1931/1961, p. 242). The purported impact of sexual abuse on a child's psyche was described in Ferenczi's 1933 work "Confusion of the Tongues Between the Adults and the Child" (Ferenczi 1949).[12] Consonant with Freud's theory, he outlined the developmental short-circuiting that takes place after abuse. In a state of confusion and overstimulation, the child, "under the pressure of such traumatic urgency [...] can develop instantaneously all the emotions of [a] mature adult" (Ferenczi 1949, p. 229). Ferenczi characterized this as "traumatic progression" or "precocious maturity." When faced with the "uninhibited, almost mad adult" (p. 229), the child is changed into a figure of premature wisdom, innocence being replaced by the false cloak of adulthood in order to survive in a world that is now unsafe.

---

[12] The 1949 date in the citation refers to the English translation by Michael Balint, published in the *International Journal of Psycho-analysis*.

Early, sustained exposure to unsafe environments can induce premature (albeit incomplete) neural circuitry development (consistent with the "stress acceleration hypothesis") (Gee et al. 2013). This may disrupt the typical timeline of neuromaturation, impacting corresponding physiological and cognitive processes. For instance, stress-induced developmental acceleration can prematurely activate memory retrieval, *shortening the infantile amnesia period* (Nielsen 2017). This underlines the child's need to pay attention to and remember aspects of the surrounding environment, given the danger it poses to survival. Individuals suffering early trauma may have vivid memories of events that took place within the first few years of life, because premature encoding was driven by the need to heighten awareness. Through this lens, infantile amnesia could be viewed as a luxury only permitted to children raised in safe-enough environments, allowing for a lowering of one's level of attention without triggering survival concerns.[13]

If traumatic experiences overwhelm one's capacities of assimilation, it will not be possible to think through the situation to gain an understanding of it (this is particularly unfathomable for a young child). Thus, other strategies will need to be deployed to make sense of adverse events and create a sense of grounding, however tenuous. This is where the defense mechanisms of turning passive into active and identification with the aggressor acquire unique relevance. One *repeats* something to avoid being at its mercy. In "Beyond the Pleasure Principle" (1920), Freud suggested that traumatic dreams may represent attempts to gain *mastery* over distressing events that might have occurred in the dreamer's past (Freud 1920/1955). (This was a departure from his earlier views on dreams as wish fulfillment, which he had posited in *The Interpretation of Dreams* [Freud 1900/1953].)

Such attempts at mastery can sometimes be observed in fragmented ways in young children. For instance, children younger than 2.5 years may respond to trauma by behaviorally reenacting aspects of the event (e.g., repetition of trauma-related movements in their play). Such behavioral dimensions are emphasized in DSM-5-TR, which outlines separate criteria for PTSD in children 6 years and younger. Examples include Criterion B3 ("trauma-specific reenactment may occur in play," p. 303) and Criterion D1 ("Irritable behavior and angry outbursts [with little or no provocation] typically ex-

---

[13] Although there is much variability, it should be noted that traumatic events per se may not be remembered with much detail or at all, which would be consistent with dissociative amnesia (i.e., loss of memory surrounding a traumatic event) and the difficulty in registering such overwhelming incidents. However, there may be memories (potentially fragmented) of *other* events from early childhood, in line with the stress acceleration hypothesis.

pressed as verbal or physical aggression toward people or objects [including extreme temper tantrums]," p. 304) (American Psychiatric Association 2022). Unconscious processing of the event is also acknowledged in the criteria, because children may have distressing dreams, either without recognizable content or with content relating to the trauma.[14]

Behavioral repetition might continue to serve as a thought substitute for processing overwhelming stimuli. Reenacting early templates, including overtly destructive components, may occur throughout life (Gobin et al. 2015; Widom 1989), including with one's peers and offspring. Experiencing emotional or physical abuse in the home has been associated with later adolescent bullying, both as perpetrator and as victim (Lucas et al. 2016). In a meta-analysis, environmental factors associated with later criminal behavior in children included home discord, childhood maltreatment, parental antisocial behavior, and child-rearing practices (Derzon 2010). Individuals with a history of early abuse or deprivation may display aggressive, unstructured, and less sensitive parenting toward their own children (Dixon et al. 2005; Dowdney et al. 1985; Ruscio 2001). More broadly, early adversity has been linked to subsequent impulsivity, affective disorders, substance use, sexual coercion, dating violence, risky sexual practices, antisocial behavior, and chronic illness and disability (Aebi et al. 2015; Felitti et al. 1998; Gunnar and Quevedo 2007; Hunt et al. 2017; Oshri et al. 2018; O'Sullivan et al. 2018; Thornberry et al. 2010; Tussey et al. 2018; Widom et al. 1995; Wilson and Widom 2008; Yampolskaya et al. 2019).

As suggested earlier, what is detrimental from a mental health standpoint might be biologically strategic to enhance fitness or reproductive success *in the short term*, an important consideration given the perils of the surrounding environment (Carter and Nguyen 2011; Srinivasan and Padmavati 1997). A shift in the timing of physiological events is exemplified by the lower age of sexual maturity observed in some women who experience early adversity, with reports of earlier menarches and increased sexual risk-taking behaviors as adolescents (Belsky et al. 2007, 2010). Of note, early menarche is associated with a concurrent acceleration in ovulatory status: if menarche occurs prior to 12 years of age, the timeline for 50% of menstrual cycles to become ovulatory is 1 year. In contrast, if menarche occurs at age 13 years or later, the same process takes *4.5 years* (Ellis 2004). From a biological standpoint, the conjunction of impulsive behaviors with earlier likelihood or chance of conception lends itself to favoring reproduction over healthier individual development, a shift driven by environmental pressures.

---

[14] Nighttime vocalizations and episodes of sleep terror have been described in traumatized children (Nielsen 2017; Terr 1988).

Women with a history of physical or sexual abuse are more likely to become pregnant during adolescence; rates of unintentional pregnancies are also higher in this population (Curry et al. 1998; Gazmararian et al. 1995; Goodwin et al. 2000; Madigan et al. 2014; Saltzman et al. 2003; Whitfield et al. 2003). Individuals with BPD (a condition associated with a very high prevalence of early abuse) can show greater promiscuity and precipitousness in entering sexual relationships (de Aquino Ferreira et al. 2018; Sansone and Sansone 2011). Critically, life expectancy in individuals with BPD can be *decreased* by up to 27.5 years (Cailhol et al. 2016; Castle 2019; Chesney et al. 2014), a *small* percentage being attributable to suicide. (BPD has been associated with medical comorbidity contributing to a shorter life span.) As such, behaviors geared toward survival may be physiologically relevant. As Belsky and Shalev (2016) stated, "[I]f contextual cues (e.g., poverty, harsh parenting, and household chaos) indicate that the environment is harsh and unpredictable, and thus infers that the future will be as well, then [programming] should accelerate development by lowering the age of sexual maturity and, thereby, increase the chance of breeding before dying, and thus passing on one's genes" (p. 1373).

The Role of Psychotherapy

Arguably, what we do in therapy is two-pronged: 1) we talk to patients, and 2) we do not overwhelm them. I will address these two deceptively simple aspects in turn, closing the neurobiological loop with a discussion of therapeutic action.

We Talk to Patients

Patients may come to treatment having maintained an eminently emotion-based understanding of self and others. If they come from traumatic backgrounds, their internal worlds might be inhabited by hateful, punitive objects, with little room for softness or relatedness. Rigidity of thinking and fixity of meaning might be the norm, sustaining immutable "truths" about oneself and the world that are not amenable to alternative perspectives. Of course, it can be a matter of psychic survival *not* to relax one's viewpoint because such a perspective might have been consolidated in the midst of overwhelming confusion and anxiety. Short-circuited approaches to the truth may have been adopted, with one clinging to whichever ready-made version of it most efficiently mitigated the distress of uncertainty. Thus, revisiting one's perspective creates the risk of reexposing oneself to such a terrifying state. The threat posed by the acquisition of further knowledge makes such an endeavor something to be attacked and avoided rather than pursued. In his discussion of the psychotic dimensions of our personalities, Bion included "a hatred of reality, internal and external, which is extended to all that makes for awareness of it" (Bion 1957, p. 266).

The neurobiological template encoded by childhood experiences may be one of heightened, maladaptive amygdala activation and stress hormone release in response to stimuli. Early negative events can shape this "default" neuroendocrine pattern, which will be "locked in" and carried forward into future interactions as a working model of relating. This can result in heightened suspiciousness and concern about the object's intentions. Therapists are no exception to these considerations, and patients may view us as being potentially just as destructive as their early objects. This lens will impact how our interventions are experienced and interpreted. For instance, patients might feel that behind our "guise" of helpful provider, there is a sadistic, exploitative monster trying to destroy them. For patients in the midst of such unsettling circumstances, the only safe haven may be the *inside of their own heads*, thus the need to be cautious about what they share with us. We invite openness and hope patients can immerse themselves in sessions, allowing their minds to drift freely from one association to the next. Yet if patients do not have a securely internalized good object, abandoning their defensive stance will not be viewed as an opportunity for productive exploration and psychic growth but rather as a potential catastrophe threatening psychic disintegration. As such, patients might be quite suspicious of us, irrespective of our good intentions. For patients, the concept of a benign object, one interested in their minds yet without malicious or selfish intent, might be very foreign. We need to be sensitive to the makeup of their internal object world and understand that any reconfiguration through psychotherapy will take time.

In the process, we may at times identify with our patients' projections and *become* the objects we are imagined to be. During sessions, we may indeed feel flustered, invaded, exhausted, or furious, among many other emotions or traits that have been assigned to a patient's internal objects. In a way, this is to be expected because patients may unconsciously try to shape the dyad into a familiar relationship model, given the perils of the unknown. When facing these pressures, sustaining a flexible, open approach to patients can help us take a step back and attempt to process the dynamic. Projective identification is, after all, a form of communication; through empathic attunement, we can experientially gain an understanding of a patient's internal object world. By remaining in contact with the emotional intensity with which a patient relates to us in sessions, we can powerfully sense, through our countertransference, the *affect-driven relational template* consolidated by the patient when interacting with objects in childhood. What was missing during those early instances was a space for empathy, and it is here that the *therapist's* VMPFC plays a crucial role. Indeed, during affectively charged moments, we might become quite rigid in our thinking, narrowing our viewpoints on patients to two-dimensional constructs and, in effect, reaffirming that no dyadic processing is possible. If we hold onto the thread of connectedness, remembering that behind acts of hostility is a desire to be found and helped, we can facilitate a model of relating that counters the internalized template of unempathic misattunement.

As mentioned, some patients come to treatment with rigid constructs of who we are, particularly if they are prone to use splitting as a defense. If the therapist turns out to be different than expected, the patient's VMPFC is recruited to make sense of the discrepancy because this cortical area is involved in updating contextual assessment after a prediction error (Wang et al. 2017). If this discrepancy can be tolerated and therapeutically processed, the therapist's mind will gain a uniqueness and value transcending the constrictions of internalized templates. As patients broaden their relational perspectives beyond part-object constructs (cf. "triangular space," discussed in Chapter 8, "The Oedipal Situation [Exclusion and Rivalry]: Theory"), the object's "otherness" will not need to be feared or effaced. Rather, a benign, interested object can be known—perhaps for the first time—and internalized into a patient's working understanding of reality. Such a progression in object awareness takes place in tandem with ever more sophisticated mentalizing abilities. The therapist's mind becomes valuable *because* of its otherness and ability to offer an independently thinking presence, one that aids in the patient's psychic growth through co-construction of meaning. In effect, *this is a transition from part-object to whole-object relating.*

In one study using psychodynamic psychotherapy for BPD (a condition commonly characterized by splitting and in which individuals may read hostile or angry intent even in neutral faces [Seitz et al. 2021]), successful treatment correlated with increased perfusion in the PFC and improvement in several clinical parameters, including self-destructive behaviors, adaptiveness of defense mechanisms, and therapeutic alliance (Lai et al. 2007). In other words, as rapport strengthens, patients are better able to modulate behavior and cognitively process distress; these improvements are facilitated by the interpersonal model of therapeutic action. As the process and mechanics of psychotherapy recruit the VMPFC of *both* therapist and patient, acquiring such clinical gains can be viewed as an instance of *internalizing the function of the good object.*[15]

Importantly, a good working alliance has been associated with better outcomes in psychotherapy (Flückiger et al. 2018; Horvath et al. 2011). In fact, there is evidence that *psychopharmacologic* agents are more effective if the alliance is strong (Cohen et al. 2017; Zilcha-Mano et al. 2015). The so-called "dodo bird verdict" posits that different modes of psychotherapy have a degree of empirical equivalence (Frank and Frank 1961; Luborsky et al. 2002); although it has garnered controversy (Carroll and Rounsaville 2010), this theory does have some level of neuroscientific support. Different forms of psychotherapy can lead to greater activation of brain areas involved with interpersonal communication and empathic attunement (e.g., VMPFC), underlining a degree of common circuitry recruitment that transcends individual modalities. This is not to invalidate the utility of certain techniques for specific conditions but rather to underline the importance of the therapeutic alliance in effecting change. This dimension should *never* be sacrificed in favor of a dogmatic allegiance to technique.

As an interesting contrast, the practice of meditation (an inherently solo endeavor) can dampen amygdala activity through an *increase* in DLPFC activation and a *decrease* in medial PFC activation. This suggests that heightening attention, cognitive control, and self-monitoring can lower autonomic response, with a neural activation pattern that is distinct from the *interpersonal* circuitry discussed previously (Brewer et al. 2011; Ives-Deliperi et al. 2011). Similar findings have been described in practitioners of mindfulness (King et al. 2016).

Over the course of psychotherapy, clinical improvement may be accompanied by a change in cortical activation patterns, with a gradual shift away from a lateral bias toward medial areas. This neurobiological transition parallels the movement toward openness and introspection patients may display with continued therapeutic work. When starting treatment, patients often bring rigid, overvalued beliefs about themselves and others, which may be driven by overly active lateral cortical areas (e.g., DLPFC) and underactive medial areas (e.g., VMPFC). Shown to be hyperactive in several psychiatric disorders, the DLPFC has been termed the "entry portal" for psychotherapy (Viamontes and Beitman 2006b). After all, this heightened activation will in-

---

[15] As a technical aside, I have found myself taking an increasingly submissive approach during sessions. I try to find a rhythm with patients, akin to a wave, calibrating my interventions not to disrupt their speech but to *synchronize* with it. Studies of conversational synchrony have highlighted the role of the VMPFC in adapting verbal output to accord with that of a conversational partner (Gordon et al. 2014). Such synchrony has been associated with prosocial behaviors, social coordination, and the establishment of rapport (Fusaroli et al. 2012). This is not to suggest that we should be talking a lot during sessions or seeking to match our patients' verbal output. Rather, we enter into the rhythm of their speech (both in its vocalizations and silences), finding ways to add our presence without being overly invasive, dominating, or overwhelming. By joining in with them in such a manner, we facilitate further expression of what is on *their* minds, beyond our own limited understanding.

form the belief patterns and cognitions that constitute the starting point of therapy. (This is aligned with the idea of "meeting patients where they are at" when initiating treatment.) As the setting becomes safe for deeper exploration, scaffolded by a sound working alliance, cognitive flexibility increases, with greater recruitment of medial cortical areas and a dampening of limbic activation (Ochsner et al. 2002; Paquette et al. 2003). These neurobiological changes have been demonstrated in major depressive disorder (MDD) with cognitive-behavioral therapy (CBT) (Goldapple et al. 2004) and interpersonal therapy (Brody et al. 2001), in PTSD with CBT (Felmingham et al. 2007; Thomaes et al. 2012), and in anxiety disorders with CBT (Furmark et al. 2002) and intensive exposure (Paquette et al. 2003; Straube et al. 2006).

Several studies have assessed the neurobiological impact of psychodynamic psychotherapy, with similar trends being observed in cortical and limbic activation, suggesting a converging therapeutic effect (Abbass et al. 2014; Marini et al. 2016). In a study of panic disorder, 4 weeks of inpatient psychodynamic treatment led to a decrease in limbic activity and an increase in ventral PFC and OFC activation (Beutel et al. 2010). After 15 months of psychodynamic therapy conducted in patients with depression, functional magnetic resonance imaging (fMRI) revealed a decrease in activation in the amygdala and in the PFC areas associated with ruminative self-referential thoughts (Buchheim et al. 2012). One case study reported the effects of 1 year of psychodynamic therapy in a patient with depression (as well as presumptive BPD), showing (on single-photon emission computed tomography [SPECT] imaging) a normalization of serotonin transporter density in the medial PFC, a metric correlating with clinical improvement (Viinamäki et al. 1998). Optimal PFC-amygdala coupling requires sufficient serotonin transporter density in the PFC, underlining the importance of this finding (Volman et al. 2013). In a study using positron emission tomography imaging, psychodynamic psychotherapy for 16 weeks was compared with the selective serotonin reuptake inhibitor fluoxetine (at dosages reaching up to 40 mg/day) for MDD (Karlsson et al. 2010). In the psychotherapy group, increased binding of the serotonin 5-HT_{1A} receptor was observed in the medial PFC and OFC, statistically separating from the medicated group and correlating with clinical improvement. 5-HT_{1A} is an inhibitory receptor subtype that decreases excitatory neurotransmission in the cortex, modulating anxiety and enhancing cortical processing. The authors correlated this serotonin effect with improvement in social functioning capacities (Karlsson et al. 2013).[16]

---

[16] The selected studies do not represent an all-inclusive list but rather serve to illustrate the objective neurobiological impact of successful psychotherapy. For a more comprehensive outline, readers are referred to the article by Miller (2017).

We Do Not Overwhelm Them

Respecting a patient's level of preparedness to engage in therapy is key to preserving the alliance and productively furthering the work. As posited by the stress inoculation hypothesis, if an individual is stressed in mild to moderate doses, within the scope of one's processing capacities, this may foster resilience and *enhance* one's ability to cope with future stressors of even greater magnitude (Edge et al. 2009; Grimm et al. 2014).

However, it can be problematic when the degree of stress exceeds the individual's cognitive capabilities. If the work of therapy causes an overwhelming fear or anxiety response, patients might prematurely abandon treatment. (In conditions such as PTSD, although psychotherapeutic interventions can be highly effective, the process of revisiting very distressing material may limit retention [Holder et al. 2019; Schottenbauer et al. 2008].) In therapy, we help patients access difficult content in a manner that allows for gradual processing. For instance, an exposure hierarchy in CBT outlines manageable, stepwise challenges that increase stress in *measured* ways, facilitating one's sense of mastery when faced with distressing circumstances. A precipitous exposure to a highly triggering cue might lead to avoidance and perpetuation of maladaptive responses.

In *Three Approaches to Psychotherapy* (Shostrom 1965) (more familiarly known as "The Gloria Films"), the founder of Gestalt therapy, Fritz Perls, referred to psychotherapy as a "safe emergency," a term reflecting both the stressful and secure nature of the work. Although we do not wish to overwhelm patients, we need to be careful not to collude with defensive avoidance of *any* difficult content. Rather, we fine-tune our interventions based on the movements within sessions, noticing when patients are able to tolerate content that is more anxiety-provoking versus when they need to move away and shut down further exploration. As we model an attuned and flexible approach, patients will allow themselves to feel increasingly vulnerable in our presence, scaffolded by our careful attentiveness.

Over time, the mind of the therapist will be valued for its presence and absence, the marker of whole-object relating. Successful treatment will strengthen cortical areas that mediate empathic attunement as well as distress tolerance. In other words, it is the *interpersonal* element of the psychotherapeutic process that enables a patient to flexibly negotiate uncertainty outside of sessions. Thus, the function of the therapist—a benign object that seeks to modify thought rather than evade it—is internalized over the course of treatment. In the process, the harshness of a patient's internal object world can be softened, allowing new modes of relating to self and others to emerge.

KEY POINTS

- Developmental neuroscience can help illustrate the internalization of working object relationship templates, in tandem with maturation of the amygdala, hippocampus, and prefrontal cortex.

- Early life adversity can result in default circuitry activation favoring a heightened stress response, leading to emotion-driven responses and a difficulty in reappraising maladaptive cognitive patterns in everyday situations.

- Effective psychotherapy can foster greater prefrontal cortex activation, with dampening of amygdala activation and improved ability to "think through" situations, including ones that might ordinarily be distressing.

- The strengthening of cortical areas associated with greater cognitive flexibility as a result of psychotherapy can be likened to an internalization of the function of the good object, modeled by the therapist.

References

Abbass AA, Nowoweiski SJ, Bernier D, et al: Review of psychodynamic psychotherapy neuroimaging studies. Psychother Psychosom 83(3):142–147, 2014 24732748

Aebi M, Landolt MA, Mueller-Pfeiffer C, et al: Testing the "sexually abused-abuser hypothesis" in adolescents: a population-based study. Arch Sex Behav 44(8):2189–2199, 2015 25981223

American Psychiatric Association: Diagnostic and Statistical Manual of Mental Disorders, 5th Edition, Text Revision. Washington, DC, American Psychiatric Association, 2022

Amodio DM, Frith CD: Meeting of minds: the medial frontal cortex and social cognition. Nat Rev Neurosci 7(4):268–277, 2006 16552413

Atzil S, Hendler T, Feldman R: Specifying the neurobiological basis of human attachment: brain, hormones, and behavior in synchronous and intrusive mothers. Neuropsychopharmacology 36(13):2603–2615, 2011 21881566

Bartels A, Zeki S: The neural correlates of maternal and romantic love. Neuroimage 21(3):1155–1166, 2004 15006682

Beebe B: Coconstructing mother-infant distress: the microsynchrony of maternal impingement and infant avoidance in the face-to-face encounter. Psychoanal Inq 20:421–440, 2000

Beebe B, Lachmann F, Markese S, et al: On the origins of disorganized attachment and internal working models: paper II. An empirical microanalysis of 4-month mother-infant interaction. Psychoanal Dialogues 22(3):352–374, 2012 23066334

Belsky J, Shalev I: Contextual adversity, telomere erosion, pubertal development, and health: two models of accelerated aging, or one? Dev Psychopathol 28(4 Pt 2):1367–1383, 2016 27688015

Belsky J, Vandell DL, Burchinal M, et al: Are there long-term effects of early child care? Child Dev 78(2):681–701, 2007 17381797

Belsky J, Steinberg L, Houts RM, Halpern-Felsher BL: The development of reproductive strategy in females: early maternal harshness –> earlier menarche –> increased sexual risk taking. Dev Psychol 46(1):120–128, 2010 20053011

Beutel ME, Stark R, Pan H, et al: Changes of brain activation pre-post short-term psychodynamic inpatient psychotherapy: an fMRI study of panic disorder patients. Psychiatry Res 184(2):96–104, 2010 20933374

Bion WR: Differentiation of the psychotic from the non-psychotic personalities. Int J Psychoanal 38(3–4):266–275, 1957 13438602

Bion W: Learning From Experience. London, Karnac, 1962

Bos K, Zeanah CH, Fox NA, et al: Psychiatric outcomes in young children with a history of institutionalization. Harv Rev Psychiatry 19(1):15–24, 2011 21250893

Brewer JA, Worhunsky PD, Gray JR, et al: Meditation experience is associated with differences in default mode network activity and connectivity. Proc Natl Acad Sci USA 108(50):20,254–20,259, 2011 22114193

Brody AL, Saxena S, Stoessel P, et al: Regional brain metabolic changes in patients with major depression treated with either paroxetine or interpersonal therapy: preliminary findings. Arch Gen Psychiatry 58(7):631–640, 2001 11448368

Buchheim A, Viviani R, Kessler H, et al: Changes in prefrontal-limbic function in major depression after 15 months of long-term psychotherapy. PLoS One 7(3):e33745, 2012 22470470

Cailhol L, Francois M, Thalamas C, et al: Is borderline personality disorder only a mental health problem? Pers Ment Health 10(4):328–336, 2016 27735136

Carroll KM, Rounsaville BJ: Perhaps it is the dodo bird verdict that should be extinct. Addiction 105(1):18–20, 2010 20078458

Carter AJ, Nguyen AQ: Antagonistic pleiotropy as a widespread mechanism for the maintenance of polymorphic disease alleles. BMC Med Genet 12:160, 2011 22151998

Castle DJ: The complexities of the borderline patient: how much more complex when considering physical health? Australas Psychiatry 27(6):552–555, 2019 31070464

Cavelzani A, Tronick E: Dyadically expanded states of consciousness and therapeutic change in the interaction between analyst and adult patient. Psychoanal Dialogues 26:599–615, 2016

Chareyron LJ, Lavenex PB, Amaral DG, Lavenex P: Postnatal development of the amygdala: a stereological study in macaque monkeys. J Comp Neurol 520(9):1965–1984, 2012 22173686

Chesney E, Goodwin GM, Fazel S: Risks of all-cause and suicide mortality in mental disorders: a meta-review. World Psychiatry 13(2):153–160, 2014 24890068

Cohen JN, Drabick DAG, Blanco C, et al: Pharmacotherapy for social anxiety disorder: interpersonal predictors of outcome and the mediating role of the working alliance. J Anxiety Disord 52:79–87, 2017 29102818

Curry MA, Perrin N, Wall E: Effects of abuse on maternal complications and birth weight in adult and adolescent women. Obstet Gynecol 92(4 Pt 1):530–534, 1998 9764624

de Aquino Ferreira LF, Queiroz Pereira FH, Neri Benevides AML, Aguiar Melo MC: Borderline personality disorder and sexual abuse: a systematic review. Psychiatry Res 262:70–77, 2018 29407572

Debiec J, Sullivan RM: The neurobiology of safety and threat learning in infancy. Neurobiol Learn Mem 143:49–58, 2017 27826033

De Brito SA, Viding E, Sebastian CL, et al: Reduced orbitofrontal and temporal grey matter in a community sample of maltreated children. J Child Psychol Psychiatry 54(1):105–112, 2013 22880630

Derzon J: The correspondence of family features with problem, aggressive, criminal, and violent behavior: a meta-analysis. J Exp Criminol 6:263–292, 2010

Dillon DG, Holmes AJ, Birk JL, et al: Childhood adversity is associated with left basal ganglia dysfunction during reward anticipation in adulthood. Biol Psychiatry 66(3):206–213, 2009 19358974

Ditzen B, Neumann ID, Bodenmann G, et al: Effects of different kinds of couple interaction on cortisol and heart rate responses to stress in women. Psychoneuroendocrinology 32(5):565–574, 2007 17499441

Dixon L, Browne K, Hamilton-Giachritsis C: Risk factors of parents abused as children: a mediational analysis of the intergenerational continuity of child maltreatment (part I). J Child Psychol Psychiatry 46(1):47–57, 2005 15660643

Dowdney L, Skuse D, Rutter M, et al: The nature and qualities of parenting provided by women raised in institutions. J Child Psychol Psychiatry 26(4):599–625, 1985 4019619

Edge MD, Ramel W, Drabant EM, et al: For better or worse? Stress inoculation effects for implicit but not explicit anxiety. Depress Anxiety 26(9):831–837, 2009 19569055

Ellis BJ: Timing of pubertal maturation in girls: an integrated life history approach. Psychol Bull 130(6):920–958, 2004 15535743

Felitti VJ, Anda RF, Nordenberg D, et al: Relationship of childhood abuse and household dysfunction to many of the leading causes of death in adults. The Adverse Childhood Experiences (ACE) Study. Am J Prev Med 14(4):245–258, 1998 9635069

Felmingham K, Kemp A, Williams L, et al: Changes in anterior cingulate and amygdala after cognitive behavior therapy of posttraumatic stress disorder. Psychol Sci 18(2):127–129, 2007 17425531

Ferenczi S: Confusion of the tongues between the adults and the child—(the language of tenderness and of passion). Int J Psychoanal 30:225–230, 1949

Flückiger C, Del Re AC, Wampold BE, Horvath AO: The alliance in adult psychotherapy: a meta-analytic synthesis. Psychotherapy (Chic) 55(4):316–340, 2018 29792475

Fonagy P, Target M: Attachment and reflective function: their role in self-organization. Dev Psychopathol 9(4):679–700, 1997 9449001

Frank JD, Frank JB: Persuasion and Healing: A Comparative Study of Psychotherapy. Baltimore, MD, Johns Hopkins University Press, 1961

Freud S: The interpretation of dreams (first part) (1900), in The Standard Edition of the Complete Psychological Works of Sigmund Freud, Vol 4. Translated and edited by Strachey J. London, Hogarth Press, 1953, pp ix–627

Freud S: Beyond the pleasure principle (1920), in The Standard Edition of the Complete Psychological Works of Sigmund Freud, Vol 18. Translated and edited by Strachey J. London, Hogarth Press, 1955, pp 1–64

Freud S: Female sexuality (1931), in The Standard Edition of the Complete Psychological Works of Sigmund Freud, Vol 21. Translated and edited by Strachey J. London, Hogarth Press, 1961, pp 221–244

Freud S: Analysis terminable and interminable (1937), in The Standard Edition of the Complete Psychological Works of Sigmund Freud, Vol 23. Translated and edited by Strachey J. London, Hogarth Press, 1964, pp 209–254

Furmark T, Tillfors M, Marteinsdottir I, et al: Common changes in cerebral blood flow in patients with social phobia treated with citalopram or cognitive-behavioral therapy. Arch Gen Psychiatry 59(5):425–433, 2002 11982446

Fusaroli R, Bahrami B, Olsen K, et al: Coming to terms: quantifying the benefits of linguistic coordination. Psychol Sci 23(8):931–939, 2012 22810169

Gabard-Durnam LJ, Flannery J, Goff B, et al: The development of human amygdala functional connectivity at rest from 4 to 23 years: a cross-sectional study. Neuroimage 95:193–207, 2014 24662579

Gazmararian JA, Adams MM, Saltzman LE, et al: The relationship between pregnancy intendedness and physical violence in mothers of newborns. Obstet Gynecol 85(6):1031–1038, 1995 7770250

Gee DG, Gabard-Durnam LJ, Flannery J, et al: Early developmental emergence of human amygdala-prefrontal connectivity after maternal deprivation. Proc Natl Acad Sci USA 110(39):15,638–15,643, 2013 24019460

Gelfo F: Does experience enhance cognitive flexibility? An overview of the evidence provided by the environmental enrichment studies. Front Behav Neurosci 13:150, 2019 31338030

Gobin RL, Reddy MK, Zlotnick C, Johnson JE: Lifetime trauma victimization and PTSD in relation to psychopathy and antisocial personality disorder in a sample of incarcerated women and men. Int J Prison Health 11(2):64–74, 2015 26062658

Goldapple K, Segal Z, Garson C, et al: Modulation of cortical-limbic pathways in major depression: treatment-specific effects of cognitive behavior therapy. Arch Gen Psychiatry 61(1):34–41, 2004 14706942

Goodwin MM, Gazmararian JA, Johnson CH, et al: Pregnancy intendedness and physical abuse around the time of pregnancy: findings from the Pregnancy Risk Assessment Monitoring System, 1996–1997. PRAMS Working Group. Pregnancy Risk Assessment Monitoring System. Matern Child Health J 4(2):85–92, 2000 10994576

Gordon RG, Tranel D, Duff MC: The physiological basis of synchronizing conversational rhythms: the role of the ventromedial prefrontal cortex. Neuropsychology 28(4):624–630, 2014 24749726

Grimm S, Pestke K, Feeser M, et al: Early life stress modulates oxytocin effects on limbic system during acute psychosocial stress. Soc Cogn Affect Neurosci 9(11):1828–1835, 2014 24478326

Gunnar MR, Donzella B: Social regulation of the cortisol levels in early human development. Psychoneuroendocrinology 27(1–2):199–220, 2002 11750779

Gunnar M, Quevedo K: The neurobiology of stress and development. Annu Rev Psychol 58:145–173, 2007 16903808

Holder N, Holliday R, Wiblin J, et al: Predictors of dropout from a randomized clinical trial of cognitive processing therapy for female veterans with military sexual trauma-related PTSD. Psychiatry Res 276:87–93, 2019 31030005

Honkaniemi J, Pelto-Huikko M, Rechardt L, et al: Colocalization of peptide and glucocorticoid receptor immunoreactivities in rat central amygdaloid nucleus. Neuroendocrinology 55(4):451–459, 1992 1373477

Horvath AO, Del Re AC, Flückiger C, Symonds D: Alliance in individual psychotherapy. Psychotherapy (Chic) 48(1):9–16, 2011 21401269

Hunt TKA, Slack KS, Berger LM: Adverse childhood experiences and behavioral problems in middle childhood. Child Abuse Negl 67:391–402, 2017 27884508

Insel TR: Is social attachment an addictive disorder? Physiol Behav 79(3):351–357, 2003 12954430

Ives-Deliperi VL, Solms M, Meintjes EM: The neural substrates of mindfulness: an fMRI investigation. Soc Neurosci 6(3):231–242, 2011 20835972

Kamphausen S, Schröder P, Maier S, et al: Medial prefrontal dysfunction and prolonged amygdala response during instructed fear processing in borderline personality disorder. World J Biol Psychiatry 14:307–318, 2013

Karlsson H, Hirvonen J, Kajander J, et al: Research letter: psychotherapy increases brain serotonin 5-HT1A receptors in patients with major depressive disorder. Psychol Med 40(3):523–528, 2010 19903365

Karlsson H, Hirvonen J, Salminen J, Hietala J: Increased serotonin receptor 1A binding in major depressive disorder after psychotherapy, but not after SSRI pharmacotherapy, is related to improved social functioning capacity. Psychother Psychosom 82(4):260–261, 2013 23736831

King AP, Block SR, Sripada RK, et al: Altered Default Mode Network (DMN) resting state functional connectivity following a mindfulness-based exposure therapy for posttraumatic stress disorder (PTSD) in combat veterans of Afghanistan and Iraq. Depress Anxiety 33(4):289–299, 2016 27038410

Knudsen EI: Sensitive periods in the development of the brain and behavior. J Cogn Neurosci 16(8):1412–1425, 2004 15509387

Kringelbach ML, Lehtonen A, Squire S, et al: A specific and rapid neural signature for parental instinct. PLoS One 3(2):e1664, 2008 18301742

Kurth F, Zilles K, Fox PT, et al: A link between the systems: functional differentiation and integration within the human insula revealed by meta-analysis. Brain Struct Funct 214(5–6):519–534, 2010 20512376

Lai C, Daini S, Calcagni ML, et al: Neural correlates of psychodynamic psychotherapy in borderline disorders—a pilot investigation. Psychother Psychosom 76(6):403–405, 2007 17917480

Lane RD, Reiman EM, Ahern GL, et al: Neuroanatomical correlates of happiness, sadness, and disgust. Am J Psychiatry 154(7):926–933, 1997 9210742

Laurent HK, Ablow JC: The missing link: mothers' neural response to infant cry related to infant attachment behaviors. Infant Behav Dev 35(4):761–772, 2012 22982277

Laurent HK, Stevens A, Ablow JC: Neural correlates of hypothalamic-pituitary-adrenal regulation of mothers with their infants. Biol Psychiatry 70(9):826–832, 2011 21783177

Lemogne C, Mayberg H, Bergouignan L, et al: Self-referential processing and the prefrontal cortex over the course of depression: a pilot study. J Affect Disord 124(1–2):196–201, 2010 19945172

Leppänen JM, Nelson CA: Tuning the developing brain to social signals of emotions. Nat Rev Neurosci 10(1):37–47, 2009 19050711

Levy J, Goldstein A, Feldman R: The neural development of empathy is sensitive to caregiving and early trauma. Nat Commun 10(1):1905, 2019 31015471

Lu Q, Li H, Luo G, et al: Impaired prefrontal-amygdala effective connectivity is responsible for the dysfunction of emotion process in major depressive disorder: a dynamic causal modeling study on MEG. Neurosci Lett 523(2):125–130, 2012 22750155

Luborsky L, Rosenthal R, Diguer L, et al: The dodo bird verdict is alive and well—mostly. Clinical Psychology: Science and Practice 9:2–12, 2002

Lucas S, Jernbro C, Tindberg Y, Janson S: Bully, bullied and abused: associations between violence at home and bullying in childhood. Scand J Public Health 44(1):27–35, 2016 26472326

Madigan S, Wade M, Tarabulsy G, et al: Association between abuse history and adolescent pregnancy: a meta-analysis. J Adolesc Health 55(2):151–159, 2014 25049043

Marini S, Di Tizio L, Dezi S, et al: The bridge between two worlds: psychoanalysis and fMRI. Rev Neurosci 27(2):219–229, 2016 26444349

McCarthy C: The kekulé problem. Nautilus, April 17, 2017. Available at: https://nautil.us/issue/47/consciousness/the-kekul-problem. Accessed July 1, 2021.

McLaughlin KA, Peverill M, Gold AL, et al: Child maltreatment and neural systems underlying emotion regulation. J Am Acad Child Adolesc Psychiatry 54(9):753–762, 2015 26299297

Milad MR, Pitman RK, Ellis CB, et al: Neurobiological basis of failure to recall extinction memory in posttraumatic stress disorder. Biol Psychiatry 66(12):1075–1082, 2009 19748076

Miller CWT: Epigenetic and neural circuitry landscape of psychotherapeutic interventions. Psychiatry J 5491812, 2017

Miller CWT: Thinking back to linking: neuroscientific correlates of Bion's theories of thought and object relating. Free Associations 19(1):65–83, 2018

Miller CWT: The impact of stress within and across generations: neuroscientific and epigenetic considerations. Harv Rev Psychiatry 29(4):303–317, 2021 34049337

Miller CWT, Ross DA, Novick AM: "Not dead yet!"—Confronting the legacy of dualism in modern psychiatry. Biol Psychiatry 87(7):e15–e17, 2020 32164918

Minzenberg MJ, Fan J, New AS, et al: Fronto-limbic dysfunction in response to facial emotion in borderline personality disorder: an event-related fMRI study. Psychiatry Res 155(3):231–243, 2007 17601709

Mizoguchi K: Ugetsu. Japan, Kadokawa Pictures, 1953

Murnane KS: Serotonin 2A receptors are a stress response system: implications for post-traumatic stress disorder. Behav Pharmacol 30(2 and 3-Spec Issue):151–162, 2019 30632995

Nejad AB, Fossati P, Lemogne C: Self-referential processing, rumination, and cortical midline structures in major depression. Front Hum Neurosci 7:666, 2013 24124416

Nelson CA III, Gabard-Durnam LJ: Early adversity and critical periods: neurodevelopmental consequences of violating the expectable environment. Trends Neurosci 43(3):133–143, 2020 32101708

Nelson CA III, Zeanah CH, Fox NA: How early experience shapes human development: the case of psychosocial deprivation. Neural Plast 2019:1676285, 2019 30774652

Nielsen T: The stress acceleration hypothesis of nightmares. Front Neurol 8:201, 2017 28620339

Ochsner KN, Bunge SA, Gross JJ, Gabrieli JD: Rethinking feelings: an FMRI study of the cognitive regulation of emotion. J Cogn Neurosci 14(8):1215–1229, 2002 12495527

Oshri A, Kogan SM, Kwon JA, et al: Impulsivity as a mechanism linking child abuse and neglect with substance use in adolescence and adulthood. Dev Psychopathol 30(2):417–435, 2018 28606210

Ostow M: Mood regulation: spontaneous and pharmacologically assisted. Neuropsychoanalysis 6:77–86, 2004

O'Sullivan D, Watts J, Shenk C: Child maltreatment severity, chronic substance abuse, and disability status. Rehabil Psychol 63(2):313–323, 2018 29878835

Paquette V, Lévesque J, Mensour B, et al: "Change the mind and you change the brain": effects of cognitive-behavioral therapy on the neural correlates of spider phobia. Neuroimage 18(2):401–409, 2003 12595193

Paré D: Role of the basolateral amygdala in memory consolidation. Prog Neurobiol 70(5):409–420, 2003 14511699

Parsons CE, Stark EA, Young KS, et al: Understanding the human parental brain: a critical role of the orbitofrontal cortex. Soc Neurosci 8(6):525–543, 2013 24171901

Paulus MP, Stein MB: An insular view of anxiety. Biol Psychiatry 60(4):383–387, 2006 16780813

Payne C, Machado CJ, Bliwise NG, Bachevalier J: Maturation of the hippocampal formation and amygdala in Macaca mulatta: a volumetric magnetic resonance imaging study. Hippocampus 20(8):922–935, 2010 19739247

Phillips ML, Young AW, Senior C, et al: A specific neural substrate for perceiving facial expressions of disgust. Nature 389(6650):495–498, 1997 9333238

Pitman RK, Rasmusson AM, Koenen KC, et al: Biological studies of post-traumatic stress disorder. Nat Rev Neurosci 13(11):769–787, 2012 23047775

Puetz VB, Parker D, Kohn N, et al: Altered brain network integrity after childhood maltreatment: a structural connectomic DTI-study. Hum Brain Mapp 38(2):855–868, 2017 27774721

Raihani NJ, Bell V: An evolutionary perspective on paranoia. Nat Hum Behav 3(2):114–121, 2019 30886903

Rountree-Harrison D, Burton TJ, Leamey CA, Sawatari A: Environmental enrichment expedites acquisition and improves flexibility on a temporal sequencing task in mice. Front Behav Neurosci 12:51, 2018 29599712

Rubin DC: The distribution of early childhood memories. Memory 8(4):265–269, 2000 10932795

Ruscio AM: Predicting the child-rearing practices of mothers sexually abused in childhood. Child Abuse Negl 25(3):369–387, 2001 11414396

Saltzman LE, Johnson CH, Gilbert BC, Goodwin MM: Physical abuse around the time of pregnancy: an examination of prevalence and risk factors in 16 states. Matern Child Health J 7(1):31–43, 2003 12710798

Sansone RA, Sansone LA: Sexual behavior in borderline personality: a review. Innov Clin Neurosci 8(2):14–18, 2011 21468292

Sapolsky RM, Meaney MJ: Maturation of the adrenocortical stress response: neuroendocrine control mechanisms and the stress hyporesponsive period. Brain Res 396(1):64–76, 1986 3011218

Schottenbauer MA, Glass CR, Arnkoff DB, et al: Nonresponse and dropout rates in outcome studies on PTSD: review and methodological considerations. Psychiatry 71(2):134–168, 2008 18573035

Schuengel C, Bakermans-Kranenburg MJ, Van IJzendoorn MH: Frightening maternal behavior linking unresolved loss and disorganized infant attachment. J Consult Clin Psychol 67(1):54–63, 1999 10028209

Seitz KI, Leitenstorfer J, Krauch M, et al: An eye-tracking study of interpersonal threat sensitivity and adverse childhood experiences in borderline personality disorder. Borderline Personal Disord Emot Dysregul 8(1):2, 2021 33397512

Shah PE, Fonagy P, Strathearn L: Is attachment transmitted across generations? The plot thickens. Clin Child Psychol Psychiatry 15(3):329–345, 2010 20603421

Sherin JE, Nemeroff CB: Post-traumatic stress disorder: the neurobiological impact of psychological trauma. Dialogues Clin Neurosci 13(3):263–278, 2011 22034143

Shin LM, Liberzon I: The neurocircuitry of fear, stress, and anxiety disorders. Neuropsychopharmacology 35(1):169–191, 2010 19625997

Shin LM, Orr SP, Carson MA, et al: Regional cerebral blood flow in the amygdala and medial prefrontal cortex during traumatic imagery in male and female Vietnam veterans with PTSD. Arch Gen Psychiatry 61(2):168–176, 2004 14757593

Shin LM, Rauch SL, Pitman RK: Amygdala, medial prefrontal cortex, and hippocampal function in PTSD. Ann N Y Acad Sci 1071:67–79, 2006 16891563

Shostrom EL: Three Approaches to Psychotherapy. Corona del Mar, CA, Psychological Films, 1965

Silbereis JC, Pochareddy S, Zhu Y, et al: The cellular and molecular landscapes of the developing human central nervous system. Neuron 89(2):248–268, 2016 26796689

Somerville LH, Kim H, Johnstone T, et al: Human amygdala responses during presentation of happy and neutral faces: correlations with state anxiety. Biol Psychiatry 55(9):897–903, 2004 15110733

Srinivasan TN, Padmavati R: Fertility and schizophrenia: evidence for increased fertility in the relatives of schizophrenic patients. Acta Psychiatr Scand 96(4):260–264, 1997 9350954

Strathearn L, Fonagy P, Amico J, Montague PR: Adult attachment predicts maternal brain and oxytocin response to infant cues. Neuropsychopharmacology 34(13):2655–2666, 2009 19710635

Straube T, Glauer M, Dilger S, et al: Effects of cognitive-behavioral therapy on brain activation in specific phobia. Neuroimage 29(1):125–135, 2006 16087353

Sullivan RM: The neurobiology of attachment to nurturing and abusive caregivers. Hastings Law J 63(6):1553–1570, 2012 24049190

Tallot L, Doyère V, Sullivan RM: Developmental emergence of fear/threat learning: neurobiology, associations and timing. Genes Brain Behav 15(1):144–154, 2016 26534899

Taylor DC: Differential rates of cerebral maturation between sexes and between hemispheres: evidence from epilepsy. Lancet 2(7612):140–142, 1969 4183249

Teicher MH, Anderson CM, Polcari A: Childhood maltreatment is associated with reduced volume in the hippocampal subfields CA3, dentate gyrus, and subiculum. Proc Natl Acad Sci U S A 109(9):E563–E572, 2012 22331913

Terr L: What happens to early memories of trauma? A study of twenty children under age five at the time of documented traumatic events. J Am Acad Child Adolesc Psychiatry 27(1):96–104, 1988 3343214

Thatcher RW, Walker RA, Giudice S: Human cerebral hemispheres develop at different rates and ages. Science 236(4805):1110–1113, 1987 3576224

Thomaes K, Dorrepaal E, Draijer N, et al: Treatment effects on insular and anterior cingulate cortex activation during classic and emotional Stroop interference in child abuse-related complex post-traumatic stress disorder. Psychol Med 42(11):2337–2349, 2012 22436595

Thornberry TP, Henry KL, Ireland TO, Smith CA: The causal impact of childhood-limited maltreatment and adolescent maltreatment on early adult adjustment. J Adolesc Health 46(4):359–365, 2010 20307825

Tottenham N, Hare TA, Millner A, et al: Elevated amygdala response to faces following early deprivation. Dev Sci 14(2):190–204, 2011 21399712

Tronick EZ, Als H, Adamson L: The structure of early face-to-face communicative interactions, in Before Speech: The Beginning of Interpersonal Communication. Edited by Bullowa M. Cambridge, UK, Cambridge University Press, 1979, pp 349–372

Tussey BE, Tyler KA, Simons LG: Poor parenting, attachment style, and dating violence perpetration among college students. J Interpers Violence 36(5–6):2097–2116, 2018 29475423

Uddin LQ, Kinnison J, Pessoa L, Anderson ML: Beyond the tripartite cognition-emotion-interoception model of the human insular cortex. J Cogn Neurosci 26(1):16–27, 2014 23937691

van IJzendoorn MH: Adult attachment representations, parental responsiveness, and infant attachment: a meta-analysis on the predictive validity of the Adult Attachment Interview. Psychol Bull 117(3):387–403, 1995 7777645

van IJzendoorn MH, Schuengel C, Bakermans-Kranenburg MJ: Disorganized attachment in early childhood: meta-analysis of precursors, concomitants, and sequelae. Dev Psychopathol 11(2):225–249, 1999 16506532

Viamontes G, Beitman B: Neural substrates of psychotherapeutic change, part I: the default brain. Psychiatr Ann 36(4):225–236, 2006a

Viamontes G, Beitman B: Neural substrates of psychotherapeutic change, part II: beyond default mode. Psychiatr Ann 36(4):238–246, 2006b

Viinamäki H, Kuikka J, Tiihonen J, Lehtonen J: Change in monoamine transporter density related to clinical recovery: a case-control study. Nord J Psychiatry 52:39–44, 1998

Volman I, Verhagen L, den Ouden HE, et al: Reduced serotonin transporter availability decreases prefrontal control of the amygdala. J Neurosci 33(21):8974–8979, 2013 23699508

Wang Y, Ma N, He X, et al: Neural substrates of updating the prediction through prediction error during decision making. Neuroimage 157:1–12, 2017 28536046

Whitfield CL, Anda RF, Dube SR, Felitti VJ: Violent childhood experiences and the risk of intimate partner violence in adults: assessment in a large health maintenance organization. J Interpers Violence 18:166–185, 2003

Widom CS: The cycle of violence. Science 244(4901):160–166, 1989 2704995

Widom CS, Ireland T, Glynn PJ: Alcohol abuse in abused and neglected children followed-up: are they at increased risk? J Stud Alcohol 56(2):207–217, 1995 7760568

Wilson HW, Widom CS: An examination of risky sexual behavior and HIV in victims of child abuse and neglect: a 30-year follow-up. Health Psychol 27(2):149–158, 2008 18377133

Yampolskaya S, Chuang E, Walker C: Trajectories of substance use among child welfare-involved youth: longitudinal associations with child maltreatment history and emotional/behavior problems. Subst Use Misuse 54(3):437–448, 2019 30658541

Zaki J, Davis JI, Ochsner KN: Overlapping activity in anterior insula during interoception and emotional experience. Neuroimage 62(1):493–499, 2012 22587900

Zeki S, Romaya JP: Neural correlates of hate. PLoS One 3(10):e3556, 2008 18958169

Zilcha-Mano S, Roose SP, Barber JP, Rutherford BR: Therapeutic alliance in antidepressant treatment: cause or effect of symptomatic levels? Psychother Psychosom 84(3):177–182, 2015 25832111

Termination

[P]sychoanalysis is no way of life. We all hope our patients will finish with us and forget us, and that they will find living itself to be the therapy that makes sense.

Donald Winnicott (1969, p. 712)

[Question]: when should analysis end?

[Bion]: it does not end; the relationship between a particular doctor and a particular analysand does.

Wilfred Bion (1990, p. 209)

In THIS FINAL CHAPTER I will discuss treatment termination. Although acknowledging there are many different perspectives on this topic, I emphasize here aspects relevant to time-limited treatment courses (e.g., in training programs) because termination is an inevitable part of the experience. In resident clinics, patients are commonly seen in psychotherapy during the outpatient year and then transferred to an incoming resident after 12 months. Sometimes there is an option to continue working with patients for an additional year. In any event, awareness of the finite nature of treatment can influence patients' engagement with the process and with the therapist, as will be discussed.

I have emphasized that in therapy, there is always an active object relationship in the room; patients will interact with us in accordance with how we are being perceived at any given moment. As discussed, shifts will occur between freely associating and shutting down communication, influencing how much access we have to a patient's mind. Allowing oneself to be vulnerable in the presence of another, no matter how benign the latter might seem,

can be challenging under the most facilitating of circumstances. This difficulty is compounded by the addition of a time limit to the treatment structure. Hence, we can understand why patients might have their walls up and
show reluctance to engage in much exploration, especially if they have just
gone through terminating with a previous resident who moved on in training or graduated. Those wounds may still be healing.

Certain markers of clinical progress have been proposed as indicators of
a patient's readiness to end treatment (e.g., enhanced ego strength, healthier
object relationships, decreased superego harshness, improved control over id-
driven impulses).[1] These goals may seem abstract and difficult to define objectively (i.e., how this might "look" in a patient). Indeed, the highly individual
nature of psychotherapy complicates overarching definitions of "treatment
success," particularly when attempting to establish common determinants
of improvement that transcend the uniqueness of each patient's experience.
If such determinants do exist, an inevitable corollary to ponder is whether
therapists should make *unilateral* decisions to end treatment, particularly if
they believe patients have achieved preestablished measures of clinical success.
Irrespective of the guidelines being followed, it is a tenuous proposition for
a therapist to state categorically that a given patient does not *need* therapy
anymore. I believe therapists should *always* involve patients in the decision-
making process of continuing, modifying, or ceasing treatment. Transition
points between providers (in residency, for instance) may be a good time to
have this conversation, because the patient and the new therapist are getting
to know each other for the first time. Some patients have remained in resident clinics for a long time, having changed therapists every 1 to 2 years. An
incoming resident may look at the patient's chart and think, "This person has
been coming here for 10 years. I don't think this patient needs to be in a residents' clinic anymore. I'm discharging the patient." Often, such short-circuited
determinations are made before the new provider has had a single session
with the patient(s) in question. This approach is profoundly invalidating of
what patients' needs might be and of what has kept them engaged in treatment all this time. We certainly would want to explore with them *why* they are
choosing a setting that requires a termination process every year or two as opposed to seeing a provider with whom they could have a longer-term relationship. Sometimes the reason is financial, because seeing a trainee is typically
associated with lower fees. However, this is not always the motivation. Train-

---

[1] In a well-known passage, Freud (1933[1932]/1964) said the intention of psycho-
analysis is "to strengthen the ego, to make it more independent of the super-ego,
to widen its field of perception and enlarge its organization, so that it can appropriate fresh portions of the id. Where id was, there ego shall be" (p. 80).

ees might imagine that *if only* particular patients had a provider who did not leave them after such a short time period, the improvements would be much greater. Yet there may be cases in which this very cycle repeats an engagement-abandonment paradigm driven by a patient's internal object organization; thus, the template is unwittingly reenacted vis-à-vis the institutional structure.[2] Plausibly, if said patient saw a provider who had an established private practice, the no-show rate might be higher; the patient might be tardy for sessions or ask to end early; there could be resistance to introspection, with marked superficiality to associations; and other dynamics might emerge that similarly underline the patient's difficulty in establishing a predictable and benign object relationship.

Patients' institutional transference can take on other forms, transcending the relationship with individual clinicians. Although providers are an important part of the therapeutic process, they are not the *whole* of it. Beyond the 50-minute meetings, the therapy experience includes all the "peripheral" elements that come before and after the actual encounter: driving that familiar route, parking in the usual space, walking up those known steps, sitting in the waiting room with its reassuring smell and décor, and reflecting afterward on what took place in the session while walking or driving away. Institutional attachment is an important component of therapy, one that precedes and survives the life span of the work with a given provider. If therapists need to be mourned, at least the structure surrounding them does not.

In other words, what patients need is *not* something we can unilaterally establish, particularly when such sweeping determinations are tethered to an incomplete understanding of their specific narratives. Rather, we must give ourselves and our patients a chance to become acquainted with one another and explore what continued work might offer. At any point in treatment (including periods of transition between providers), the decision to stop therapy should be made *with* the patient, not on our own.[3] The use of "objective markers" to signal that the work of psychotherapy has unquestionably run its course and that continuing it would be futile may well represent a rationalization on our part to end treatment with someone we find inconvenient or frustrating; in such instances, it will be important to assess our countertransference and reflect on what is being reenacted with this par-

---

[2] Cf. the discussion of John Bowlby's theory in Chapter 6. As I indicated there, selection of certain environments by an individual may be a way of reinforcing internalized modes of relating in accordance with working models (see Bowlby 1973).

[3] Ferenczi (1927/1994) stated, "The proper ending of an analysis is when neither the physician nor the patient puts an end to it, but when it dies of exhaustion, so to speak. (...) A truly cured patient frees himself from analysis slowly but surely; so long as he wishes to come to analysis, he should continue to do so" (p. 85).

ticular patient. If we find ourselves strongly wanting to discharge someone, we should take a step back, discuss the case with a supervisor, and find a way to productively address the situation with the patient.

Once termination is concretely on the horizon, patient-therapist dynamics may change considerably. By signifying the end of the relationship, termination carries a weight and relevance that transcend modality, frequency, and duration of treatment. The most well analyzed patient can be deeply unsettled by the termination process, leading to unanticipated and potentially problematic responses. How a patient will experience the end of the therapeutic relationship can never be reliably predicted; it must be *lived through* to become known. As Orens (1955) observed, "The threat of separation from the analysis caused a flow of previously unknown material, and deeper levels of the unconscious were uncovered" (p. 664).

As termination is navigated, therapeutic gains from preceding sessions will not necessarily inoculate patients against feelings of grief or betrayal. Strong, often maladaptive defense mechanisms can be summoned to soften the blow. A clinician might view such developments as disheartening indicators of treatment failure, underestimating the meaning and impact of the work done thus far. Yet it is important to maintain an overarching perspective of the treatment, recognizing its successes while respecting the patient's need to ease the pain by resorting to defensive measures. It is often *because* the therapy has been so significant that its loss is felt so deeply, leading to strong reactions in the patient. Keeping this viewpoint in mind can help the therapist feel grounded and retain a sense of value.

The impact of termination on the *therapist* also needs to be considered. Over the course of treatment, we become attached to our patients. We learn intimate details about their lives, think about them between sessions, discuss them with colleagues and supervisors, and look forward to meeting with them from week to week. Indeed, our interactions with them can add to a sense of predictability and comfort in *our* lives. As a result, we too will need to mourn the loss of the therapeutic relationship and expect potential shifts in how we interact with our patients during the final stages of treatment. Lafarge (2019) stated, "As termination approaches, the analyst is confronted with less accessible countertransferences" (p. 1283).[4]

In the following sections, I will further my discussion on how patient and provider are impacted by the loss of the relationship. Given the targeted scope of this chapter, I will not be discussing how to gauge clinical readiness

---

[4] Orgel (2000) has pointed out some of the therapist's struggles in working through termination, stating, "We must face the fact that in the termination period regressive pulls often exert their greatest strength in the analyst" (p. 733).

or suitability for ending treatment; I refer interested readers to select works addressing these dimensions (Freud 1937/1964; Gabbard 2009; Klein 1950; Lafarge 2019; Lussana 2018; Orgel 2000).

Beginning, Ending, and Beginning Again

Within the clinic structure of some programs, junior trainees take the place of graduating ones at the turn of the academic calendar. Thus, for a given patient, the grieving of one relationship is followed by immediate engagement in another.[5] At the beginning of the academic year, trainees are often quite enthusiastic to start working with the patients they "inherited." Yet this enthusiasm can be significantly dampened by a puzzling *lack* of commitment on the patients' part. Some patients will simply not answer or return calls for an initial appointment. Others will respond, but only to indicate they are dropping out of treatment. For patients who do return, some might express a wish to "convert" to more problem-oriented therapy or to medication management. Some patients, of course, will wish to continue psychodynamic work with the incoming provider. Yet a seamless reengagement is far from the norm. Rather, there may be considerable reluctance to open up to the new therapist, with limited associations and prolonged silences during sessions.

As we try to make sense of these varied responses from our patients, it is important to remember that they might still be grieving a relationship with a previous provider, which may have ended as recently as the week or month prior. Twelve months ago, their therapeutic journey began with someone different, under circumstances that were conspicuously similar to the present ones. A space for closeness and joint exploration was gradually fostered, allowing for new depths in self-understanding to be accessed. Yet these therapeutic gains do not eliminate the verdict imposed by reality: the relationship has ended.[6] What a new therapist is implicitly proposing, alongside any possible clinical benefits, is a revisiting of this mourning process in 1–2 years. Un-

---

[5] Although it may feel there is something artificial to this structure, it is not that far removed from realities outside of training settings. A course of psychotherapy can be short-lived or prematurely interrupted for a variety of reasons, such as a change in therapist or patient availability (because of job, schedule, or personal demands on either part, including retirement by the provider), an increase in session fees or changes in insurance coverage (making continuation inviable), therapist or patient relocation, and loss of employment or source of income by the patient, among countless others. Experiences with previous providers will inevitably influence a patient's ability to recommit to the process with a new therapist, regardless of setting.

[6] Cf. Freud's observations regarding the mourning process, noting that one's "attachment to the lost object is met by the verdict of reality that the object no longer exists" (Freud 1917[1915]/1957, p. 255).

derstandably, patients might not be too keen to re-create a relationship with the potential for such anguish at its end point. Thus, a patient may defend against establishing the same level of relatedness with the incoming provider. At times, this takes the form of overly idealizing or devaluing the previous therapist, sessions being filled with observations and ruminations about the former provider. While such a focus will be important in processing the recent loss, becoming overly and persistently fixated on the prior therapist can serve to *keep out* the new one. The latter is not allowed an individual, worthwhile presence within the dyad, being relegated to living in the shadow of the predecessor. This leaves the new therapist feeling just as excluded as the patient may have felt at the hands of the departing trainee.

Although this barrier can be frustrating, it is therapeutically useful to empathize with our patients' need to keep us from coming too close, lest they risk grieving another loss down the line. However, we can also wonder with them if the success of the previous treatment was *entirely* contingent on the therapist. If not, what was it that *the patient* brought to sessions that allowed the work to be meaningful? What aspects within the patient were strengthened by the previous therapy, and how can we make them accessible to be built upon further, even if the provider is different? The end of a relationship does not signify the end of individual progress. The very fact that patients *choose to remain* in treatment, despite trepidation and sadness, suggests that, on some level, they feel capable of productively engaging with the new therapist and continuing the work.

Alternatively, there are patients who seem *immediately* ready to pick up where they left off. During transition of care, the graduating provider might report to the incoming trainee that some patients "handled termination wonderfully, as though they didn't even care I was leaving." When the new therapist meets them, they may be gregarious, enthusiastic, and willing to speak without hesitation about deeply personal issues. The therapist might feel "welcomed" by such a form of engagement. Accompanying this, however, is the unsettling sense that the patient is viewing whoever happens to be sitting across the room as entirely generic and replaceable, with no individual staying power to speak of. Far from being a whole object with nuanced and unique traits, the therapist becomes a part-object, a carbon copy of the one before and likely of the one to follow. Just as the therapist was readily "taken up" at the beginning of treatment, termination may be handled with the same "ease," 12 months later (akin to what was described with the previous provider). In such instances, the patient will divest the impending end of any greater meaning, focusing primarily on the mechanics of the transition. (In other words, as long as the patient is seen by *someone* after termination, there is nothing else to discuss.) This is conceptually important, because the defenses and interpersonal dynamics observed at the beginning of treatment can re-emerge toward its end. The therapist's place as a unique, valued object is de-nied—the relationship going in is ready-made, impersonal, and two-dimensional. If no dependence is fostered, grief can be averted when the time comes to part ways. Even if important work has been done over the course of treatment, the significance of the relationship may be gradually dismissed as the termination date draws closer.

Negotiating the beginning of a therapeutic process can be difficult even when defenses are less overt. There is something very appealing about reach-ing the "middle phase" of therapy, when a certain rhythm to sessions has been established. Factors contributing to this include the regularity of the meeting time, an understanding and observance of the frame, and an implicit awareness within the dyad of how the other operates over the course of a given hour. For both patient and therapist, these aspects confer a level of familiar-ity, predictability, and comfort to the proceedings. In the midst of stressful and unpredictable lives, regular therapy sessions may be the only stable, grounding routine patients have.

While this dynamic might seem desirable and comforting, it may not be *allowed* to take form, particularly if one's internal object world repudiates the existence of such a relational construct. In such cases, patients might repel at-tempts by the therapist to become a predictable object. One method of doing so is by impinging on the frame. (While I have discussed the frame at length in an earlier chapter [see Chapter 3: "Establishing and Maintaining a Ther-apeutic Frame"], I will return to the topic briefly to highlight its relevance in termination.) Patients might try to shift appointment times from week to week, arrive late to sessions (tardiness sometimes varying from one session to the next, ensuring there is no regularity *even to their lateness*), or occasionally not show up. In such instances, the frame becomes little more than a theo-retical construct. Discussing the meaning of breaks or termination seems al-most absurd, given the shifting ground on which the relationship was built. However, handling the frame in such a manner can serve an important com-municative function. It may, for instance, reflect internalized relationship tem-plates in which early objects were unpredictable and noncontaining, leaving the child in a state of unmitigated distress. Through projective identification (effected by the patient's repeated frame violations), the therapist *becomes* this inconsistently available figure who is unable to make proper sense of the patient's mind, a recasting of the internal object who never established itself as reliably present.

Hopefully, this will be noticed and discussed with patients. For instance, we can wonder with them what it would mean if they were to show up on time and have regular appointments each week. This would, if nothing else, position the therapist as a *different* type of object from the internalized one, with attempts to access and understand the patient's inner world replacing the mindless reliving of damaging templates. However, if the therapist is allowed a place of uniqueness, this creates the potential for dependence and eventual grief when the work ends. As a result, attempts to explore the significance of the frame impingements may be met with dismissiveness or resistance. After all, if we are not allowed to acquire importance as meaningful objects, we will not pose a threat to the patient's internal object constructs, nor will we need to be mourned as worthy objects in our own right.[7]

Bringing Up Termination: The Therapist's Role and Reaction

Discussions regarding termination should occur when there is sufficient time to process it. If it is known beforehand that treatment will be ending (e.g., in training settings), (re)introducing the topic at least a few months before the final session is recommended. It is also useful to set a concrete termination date and hold to it. (A joint decision should be made about when to have the last session.) As the end draws near, the therapist, patient, or both might feel tempted to push the stop date to a later time, perhaps to delay experiencing the loss. However, this should be avoided as much as possible. Reality is only optional up to a certain point, and part of establishing ourselves as reliable objects is acknowledging the limits of our availability rather than yielding to manic urges to bend time. Though painful, mourning the relationship is part of the therapeutic journey, and a space for the grieving process to unfold must be fostered. By shifting the stop date, we are dislodging the *necessary* reference point around which the work of termination orbits, unmooring the dyad from the delicate working-through required for healthy transitioning.

---

[7] These considerations argue for the importance of maintaining a regular meeting time with patients, as opposed to shifting from one week to the next. The specific timeslot shared by patient and therapist becomes increasingly meaningful the more it is preserved. Critically, the significance of the frame can only be understood and interpreted *if the frame is allowed to exist.* When a session does not take place during a given week (e.g., with vacation or illness), we can explore how that hour, now consistently associated with therapy, was experienced by the patient. Perhaps the patient felt pangs of loneliness, cold, dread, fear, sleepiness, indifference, or some other emotional or somatic response. These might represent reactions to the lack of the physicality or sensorial qualities of the therapeutic space; although wishing to immerse oneself into that familiar room with a welcoming therapist, it was unavailable, and the "void" was felt viscerally.

We need to be empathic to *ourselves*, too. We may have unexpected emotional reactions to losing contact with patients we have come to value greatly, people who were active participants in shaping our professional identity and furthering our competency. Termination can feel like a large-scale recapitulation of individual session dynamics: we are present and welcoming for a while; then we are gone. The guilt experienced over such "deprivation" (particularly if a rise in professional status is awaiting us after our departure) can lead us to deny or minimize our importance to patients. A graduating clinician may veer termination discussions toward the logistical aspects of the transition, emphasizing the attributes of the incoming provider, focusing on medication refills, and letting the patient know when to expect a call from the new therapist. Meanwhile, the real and irreplaceable loss going on in the lives of the two individuals *presently* in the room is ignored. Therapists may turn themselves into depersonalized clinicians in training or mere prescribers, dismissing their own individuality and the unique role they played in their patients' psychic growth. This stance eliminates the need to process the end of the relationship.

I tell residents that discussing the logistics of transitioning care does not need to occupy more than a few minutes in session, especially if the structure of the clinic is largely unchanging and if the patient has been through the process before. While the finer details will vary depending on the specifics of each case, the practical aspects of the transition can be encapsulated by the following: "As of July 1, a new therapist will be taking my place at the clinic. I'll let you know the name as soon as I have that information; you can expect a call within the first few weeks of July. I'll be sure to prescribe enough medication so you don't run out." The rest of the termination discussion should focus on the *current* relationship and how the patient feels about its forthcoming end. The therapeutic space being lost is one that has been carefully nurtured by the dyad over the preceding months or years, and minimizing its importance cheats it of its value. We also need to give ourselves a chance to feel a sense of accomplishment with the patient for the work that has been done. Whatever the gifts of the incoming therapist may be, we are *not* interchangeable. The place we hold in our patients' lives, and what it means to lose us, will be highly unique. In a year or two, the patient can reflect on how wonderful the next therapist was, but now is *our* time.

The Patient's Experience of Termination

It has often been observed that the termination of an analysis reactivates in the patient earlier situations of parting, and is in the nature of a weaning experience. This implies, as my work has shown me, that the emotions felt by the baby at weaning time, when early infantile conflicts come to a head, are strongly revived towards the end of an analysis. (Klein 1950, p. 78)

Even if the time-limited aspect of treatment was raised at the beginning of the work, when the time comes to discuss the reality of terminating, patients can feel quite ill prepared. They may have hoped that their therapists' training would be extended or that they could follow the graduating providers to their next practice setting. The patient might feel abandoned, unimportant, or like a mere stepping-stone for the therapist to complete training before moving on to treat a more "worthwhile" clientele.

Although we hope to provide a benign model of curiosity and kindness, our purported "good object–ness" can become soured when the reality that treatment will end is increasingly brought into focus. Compounding this is the inescapable aliquot of *truth* to the idea that we are leaving our patients to further our own pursuits, often continuing our journey in settings that pay more and confer greater prestige.[8] Although training in order to master one's craft is part and parcel of professional development, this is cold comfort to patients who have worked hard to co-construct the therapeutic space, allowing themselves to experience vulnerability in the presence of a trusted object.

As briefly discussed in an earlier section, defenses can be mounted to lessen the impact of the loss. For instance, patients might deny there ever *was* any importance to the relationship. The part of themselves that felt connected to the therapist and invested in the work may be projected into the provider, who becomes the only one assigning meaning to the relationship. A therapist who asks how a patient is feeling about the end might be answered with, "You always think you're so important. You ask about breaks between sessions, holidays, weekends, and now the end of therapy. You don't live with me outside of this room. I only see you for an hour each week. You're not *that* important. I feel *nothing* when there are breaks, and I feel *nothing* about ending

---

[8] These considerations extend beyond structural logistics outside the therapist's control. Sometimes trainees do have the option of carrying forward select patients for an additional year. Some patients do not "make the cut," and the trainee might feel guilty for favoring one over the other. Rationalized arguments may posit that the chosen patients were the ones offering the "best learning opportunities," when in fact likability carried the greatest weight. Gabbard (2009) noted, "Perhaps one of the greatest psychoanalytic myths of termination is that the assessment of readiness is based on a set of criteria that do not take the analyst's self-interest into account" (p. 588). How much and for how long a therapist interacts with patients may be strongly influenced by one's degree of tolerance for them. Providers should be very mindful of the potential for destructive reenactments stemming from countertransference dislike and impatience. This consideration is not something to be shrugged off but rather needs to be taken quite seriously, given its potential to adversely impact how one treats a patient who is suffering and coming to therapy for help.

therapy." Met with such a response, therapists may feel silly for having brought it up, thinking perhaps they *are* making too much of themselves. However, this might be how projective identification is taking form. When faced with the potential for loss and grief, patients can reclaim a sense of control by pushing the needy, dependent, "I care about therapy" trait onto the provider, whose insistence on discussing termination may fuel the patients' sense that they themselves are the ones worthy of being missed, while the therapist is turned into someone disposable. A spoiled object is not needed, nor does it deserve to be mourned.

Feelings of envy can inform a need to devalue the therapist, whose departure suggests the provider has become "too good" to treat "training cases." While the therapist moves on to a special, privileged life, patients are stuck in the mire of ordinary existence, dealing with some of the same struggles they had when therapy started. When the push to devalue is present, it can be difficult to hold onto the thread of relatedness and acknowledge that real improvements *have* taken place, as much as they are being defensively minimized. One way to reassure oneself that therapy is not needed is to "convince" both parties that the time together made absolutely no difference, thus erasing any psychic footprints the therapist might have left. Indeed, patients may argue that things have gotten *worse* and that the therapist actually did them harm. A feeling of triumph, anger, or indifference toward the therapist can be preferable to grief.

Alternatively, facing termination might cause patients to strongly *idealize* the therapist. The latter becomes the repository of a patient's capacity for self-reflection and continued psychic growth. Without the therapist, the patient can feel untethered and at risk of destructive setbacks. When termination is broached, patients may despair at the "news," saying they had been hoping against hope this day would never arrive, having fantasized about some magical loophole that could allow the work to continue. They might tell the therapist quite directly how cruel it is to be abandoning them, stating, "I've never opened up like this to anyone before. I cannot start over with someone new. If I can't see you, I *refuse* to see anyone else. You might as well just discharge me if we can't keep doing therapy together."

If the therapist identifies as the sole catalyst for change, tremendous guilt can result. The therapist may indeed forget that the *patient* did a great deal of work in therapy all along and that clinical gains were only possible because of *both minds* in the room. Under such pressures, this perspective can become lost, the treatment narrative being fiercely telescoped into this act of "treason" by the therapist. Such dynamics reflect the regressive pull on patient and therapist, both identified as part of a primitive couple with impossibly asymmetric powers. Within it, the therapist is psychically holding onto an exceptionally fragile creature; any movement risks shattering it into tiny pieces. As Orgel (2000) stated,

> On the most primitive level, the analysand, when most immersed in regression, may have had to believe he or she would merge with, and possess forever, the life-sustaining power attributed to the analyst, an illusion that the analyst is like the earliest parental imago, whose presence restores a sense of wholeness when overwhelming instinctual demands threaten disintegration and chaos. (p. 733)

This form of relating is reminiscent of early development in the paranoid-schizoid position, as discussed in Chapter 6 ("Developing a Sense of Self: Theory"; see section "Klein and the Paranoid-Schizoid Position"). Just as bad/hostile aspects of the self can be projected into an object (which is then seen as persecutory), projection of one's *good* traits can take place, conferring all-good and life-sustaining properties to the object. This is a normal developmental process. Indeed, the containing object will show itself to be positively affected by the child's gestures. The child will thus experience the self as possessing worthwhile, loving qualities. These affirming interactions will allow the child to re-introject and take ownership for the good aspects of the self, knowing one has a positive, affiliative impact on others. However, this process can also go awry, with notable implications. Per Klein (1946),

> The projection of good feelings and good parts of the self into the mother is essential for the infant's ability to develop good object relations and to integrate his ego. However, if this projective process is carried out excessively, good parts of the personality are felt to be lost [...]; this process, too, results in weakening and impoverishing the ego. Very soon such processes extend to other people, and the result may be an extreme dependence on these external representatives of the good parts of the self. (pp. 102–103)

If a child's inner world is overly occupied by distressing, hateful internal objects, it may feel that the latter will ruin *any* good the self contains. As a protective measure, one's good traits will be projected into the object "for safekeeping" (Boyer 1978, p. 68), lest the self's inner destructiveness erase them.[9] Thus, the individual will not view the self as possessing inherently positive, growth-promoting abilities, because the idealized object has become (through projection) the only source of goodness and stability. In the scenario outlined earlier, a regressive movement in therapy takes place wherein the patient feels

---

[9] Individuals with a trauma history may view the self as inherently toxic or damaged, with little remaining of an inherent sense of value or worth.

that any chance of psychic survival depends entirely on the continued physical presence of the all-good therapist.[10]

It will be part of the working-through of termination to notice these strong reactions by patients while avoiding collusive identification as the all-bad or all-good object. Termination is *not* an annihilating reality, nor are we messianic agents who can right all wrongs in a patient's life. Rather, it is important to empathize with the distress caused by the reality of the situation but also to remind the patient that *both* members of the dyad played a part in reaching moments of greater truth and relatedness. Whatever was strengthened in the patient's mind through therapy will remain active and capable of furthering the work, even without the therapist's presence.

To maintain this perspective, we need to keep *ourselves* grounded in the larger narrative of the work. By doing so, we can recognize these oscillations away from the depressive position for what they are: oscillations. Although it can be difficult to reach patients operating in paranoid-schizoid modes, the need for such fluctuations must be respected. We may transiently need to hold onto feelings of incompetence, uselessness, or guilt in order to help patients experience a greater sense of control over this very challenging situation. This is the value of "wearing the patient's attributions" to empathically further exploration in the midst of difficult transference dynamics (Lichtenberg 1998). It is important not to fully identify with the projection, but it is crucial not to defensively cast it off. We may feel quite unsettled by the thanklessness of the dynamic, having the urge to say, "I am *too* helpful! You *are* feeling better! You *will too* miss me!" In effect, we would have to *aggressively* affirm to patients just how benevolent we are, kindness paradoxically being expressed through hostility. It might make it *that much easier* for patients to leave us behind if our most valued qualities have been sullied. We need to trust the sturdiness of the relationship to weather these storms, maintaining our empathic stance and noticing moments when patients are psychically available to discuss termination in less defended ways.

Of course, processing the vicissitudes of termination is only possible if patients continue to attend sessions until the stop date. This is not always the case, because patients may choose to end therapy early, on their own terms. As a sense of self-sufficiency is shored up, patients might dismiss the utility of continuing work with someone whose availability is so limited. Instead of just watching the sand run through the hourglass set in front of them, they set *their own* on the table, one with a much wider neck. By claiming some

---

[10] Given the impossibility of conforming to idealizing pressures and the inevitability of termination, the therapist can quickly become the persecutory, all-bad object (i.e., the converse of the idealized object).

control over arguably the most important component of the frame (i.e., whether therapy happens or not), they can negotiate the inevitability of separateness in a way that gives them the abandoning rights. Indeed, *we* may then be left feeling even more guilty and grief-stricken, having planned to work through this difficult situation for our patients' benefit *as well as our own*. When this processing is interrupted by a premature termination, we might wonder what we could have done differently to keep the patient from leaving (a question patients may have asked *themselves* when confronted with the reality of *our* departure).

When patients suddenly stop coming or say they wish to call it quits before the final scheduled session, it is not usually helpful to exhort them repeatedly to return. After missed sessions, we can place one or two calls to indicate we are available and hopeful they will return for the remaining appointments. (Note that if there are safety concerns, we need to take more proactive steps to ensure the patient is not at risk.) It is not recommended to leave extensive voice messages or send long emails elaborating on content discussed in session in the hopes of drawing the patient back. Therapy is a two-person process and cannot be done when one party is absent. While we wait for a response from our patients, we keep ourselves open to the possibility of their return when they are ready while also acknowledging this might not happen.

A woman I worked with for 2 years in twice-weekly treatment informed me she would be relocating for family reasons in a few months. We set a date for our final session. She continued to show up regularly, with termination at the forefront of our discussions. Her distress became increasingly palpable as the weeks progressed. With 1 month remaining until our stop date, she told me at the end of a session that her work schedule was going to be slightly different for the remaining weeks before her move and that she would have to get back to me about alternative appointment times. She left the session with neither of us knowing when the next one would be. A week went by with no contact. I called her. (Over the preceding 2 years, she had *never* failed to answer the phone when I called.) She did not pick up. I left a message saying I looked forward to hearing from her about resuming sessions. Nothing. Another week went by. I left another message, admittedly with more affect, saying it was very important for us to discuss what was happening and that I hoped she would return my call. We never met or spoke again. However, around 1 year later, I received a letter from her. She described how painful it was to be losing me and that she did not know how else to terminate other than to remove me from her life completely. She wrote, "It was the only way to stop my soul from bleeding." She thanked me and said she had started therapy with another provider in her new town.

As I read her powerful words, I found myself evocatively reflecting on the oft-told narrative of how some individuals on their deathbeds eventually pass. While surrounded by family and friends, they may hold onto life, even if they are very ill. At some point, they may instruct their loved ones to go rest, run an errand, or do something otherwise trivial that would remove them from the room. Once physically alone, they allow themselves to die. This underlines an existential need to negotiate the ultimate separateness on their own terms. Reality dictates the end of our lives and, in many cases, the end of therapeutic relationships as well. We cannot expect people to unquestioningly allow their vulnerability to be shared with or witnessed by someone healthier who will go on living without them.

Clinical Vignette

Mr. R was a single 50-year-old man with whom I had worked in therapy for 3 years. Because of an unexpected change in his job demands, we needed to plan for termination with only 2 months' notice. Our work had revolved largely around his difficulty forming close relationships, given his guardedness with others and fear of "losing himself" in the emotional whirlpool of intimacy. I learned about many "false starts" in his dating life, his checklists of required attributes in a partner, and the various ways in which he would "ghost" his dates (i.e., cease communication with them entirely and without notice) when he did not think they were compatible.

While his parents were minimally involved in his upbringing, his grandmother had been a central figure during his early childhood. She died when Mr. R was 7 years old. He described this loss as utterly devastating, feeling his "life compass" had been snatched away. In later relationships, Mr. R had great difficulties allowing intimacy to develop, worrying that closeness might expose the "gaping childhood wound" left by his grandmother's death. His career became the organizing aspect of his life, though he found little satisfaction in it.

As we approached the termination date, themes of loss, death, and unresolved grief started to emerge in his associations. (Of note, prior to our final sessions, Mr. R had not shared how significant his grandmother had been to him, nor had he spoken of how profoundly her death had affected him.) In our penultimate session, he told me about an incident that occurred when he was on vacation in Western Europe. Mr. R was driving his rental car on the expressway and noticed a man on a bicycle around half a mile down the road. The man was preparing to rush across the expressway instead of using the overpass and attempted to do so just as Mr. R was approaching his location. Mr. R saw the man crossing and desperately put on the brakes, but there was no way to swerve or slow down in time. He ran into the man at almost full speed. As Mr. R pulled over and got out of the car, a crowd of spectators gathered. He began pleading for someone to help because he was clearly shaken up and could not find his phone. (It had been sitting on the passenger seat and was propelled out of reach by the crash.) To his despair and confusion, no one took any initiative to call for an ambulance or to help the injured man on the road. Mr. R ran to a public phone to call the police. When they arrived, the officers were quite nonchalant about the situation and calmly walked with Mr. R to the accident scene. One of the officers dragged the man's body off the road and rolled him into the thicket to the side of the expressway. Mr. R angrily cried out, "What are you *doing*? We need an *ambulance*!" The officer responded coolly, "An ambulance? For what? Dude's dead." At this point in the session, Mr. R looked up at me and said, "I knew he wasn't dead. Something could have been done...." He finished the account, telling me paramedics eventually arrived at the scene and immediately pronounced the man dead. Mr. R fell silent after recounting this. I had remained quiet throughout his hypnotizing narrative. An encroaching sense of terror had slowly taken over me as I pictured the events he was describing.

Suddenly, his attire and demeanor came into sharp focus. Mr. R typically dressed in bright, vibrant colors. He was quite gregarious and smiled frequently during sessions. This time, however, his clothes were dark and muted. He appeared defeated as he spoke, slouching in the chair and making poor eye contact. He stated, "I remember my grandmother dying.... She was in her bed....I was sitting next to her, crying my eyes out. Someone told me suddenly, 'She's gone.' I didn't say anything for days after that. What was there to say? Death has the final word in everyone's story."

He then told me he had stopped taking his antidepressant for the past week, even though it had been very helpful. He was slowly letting go of me and of anything I could offer him, even if doing so proved harmful. Throughout the session, I noticed a resistance within *myself* to explore the deeper meaning of what Mr. R was telling me. It seemed I was colluding with the idea that there was nothing salvageable between us. He had risked crossing the dangerous expressway of therapy, fostering a closeness that might expose his "gaping childhood wound." Termination had hit him, and we were both struggling to determine whether something between us remained alive or if we should pronounce the therapy dead.

As I attempted to recover my mind, I told him simply, "It's hard for you to lose me." He gave me a bewildered look, one I had never seen before, as though we were both losing our grip on reality. After a minute of silence, he stated numbly, "Living...is very difficult." I told him, "It's very challenging not to see despair all around. Yet there's a part of you still *very much* alive and capable of moving forward with the growth you obtained during therapy." He stared at the floor as I said this. Time was up. For the first time in 3 years, he left without shaking my hand.

When Mr. R came back for our last session, the dynamic was strikingly different. He was dressed in *very* bright colors. Throughout the encounter, he spoke quite loudly and laughed frequently. He began by telling me, "I feel amazing. I'm ready to take on life after therapy." He laughed. "I don't think we need to talk about last session at all." I felt he had donned a thick armor and that anything I had to contribute would be ricocheted right back. Our swan song was marked by this manic flight into health, a defensive response to the grief he had experienced during the previous meeting. Acknowledging his need for me confronted him with a pain too terrible to endure. He asked me if I knew any supportive therapists, "someone to problem solve with." He stated, "I think I'm done with this deep, 'digging up the past' hocus-pocus." My surprise gradually turned into annoyance. I found myself thinking perhaps he *would* be better off with a different type of therapist and that *both of us* benefited from the termination. Evidently, our respective defenses were being summoned to deal with the impending separation. I was telling myself (as Mr. R was telling *himself*) that the end of the relationship was not a big deal and that we would do just fine (perhaps *better*) without one another. As Gabbard (2009) indicated, "The impending loss through termination not uncommonly mobilizes manic defenses in both parties to deny loss" (p. 588).

Mr. R then said, "Never mind. I can find a therapist on my own." While I gave him a list of therapists anyway (which he took from me unenthusiastically), I never found out if he reengaged in treatment. Because he had stopped his medication, he did not even want a prescription from me. I tried hard to remind myself that this last session did not tell the whole story. Yet I remained haunted by the unnerving feeling that I had been ghosted.

Finding a Way Forward

[The course the analyst must pursue] is one for which there is no model in real life.

Sigmund Freud (1915/1953, p. 163)

The work of termination, like other kinds of mourning, entails the working through of the paranoid-schizoid phantasies that have emerged and a return to the depressive position, with the good object, lost in external reality, now installed in psychic reality.

Lucy Lafarge (2019, p. 1272)

Just as all treatment courses are unique, the same can be said for the process of termination. As suggested by the Bion quote at the beginning of this chapter, the work of self-exploration and psychic healing does not end with the cessation of sessions. Patients' lives will go on after we part ways, yet something of us will remain with them, whether or not they engage with another therapist in the future. Over the arc of treatment, we facilitate an emotionally intimate process that inevitably must end. Mourning this loss can be difficult, but hopefully our presence will be registered as a new type of internal object, one that is benignly invested in the patients' psychic development. This reconfiguration in one's internal object world, promoted by the therapeutic process, opens space and creates the scaffolding required for continued psychic growth.

This optimal outcome does not always line up with the reality of termination, which can be quite anticlimactic. However, even if the final sessions are unsatisfying to one or both parties, we should not lose sight of the moments of attunement and healing that took place over the course of therapy. Such instances remain invaluable despite the defensive pull toward omnipotence and devaluing when confronting loss. It is important to view termination as a *working-through* process. At times, there may be a stepwise progression in dynamics similar to those outlined by Steiner in his breakdown of the depressive position (Steiner 1992) (see Chapter 9, "The Oedipal Situation [Exclusion and Rivalry]: Clinical"). In the first substage, when "fear of loss of the object" predominates, separateness can be effaced through attempts to identify with the object. Patients may try to find *some* way of keeping the therapist in their lives. For instance, if the provider is going into private practice after graduating, patients might strongly insist on continuing treatment at the new location, even if this entails moving or paying a much higher fee. Through identification, the patient joins in the therapist's "ascent": just as the therapist is becoming someone "important" who can *charge* more, the patient is also elevated to a new status and is suddenly able to *pay* more. (Whether or not this ability is based in reality is a separate matter; what is notable is the deployment of defenses through which the patient is lifted above the ordinary status of a "droppable" training case.)

The next substage is "experience of loss of the object," requiring one to acknowledge separateness and let go of the object. As termination is lived through, we hope patients can grieve us and continue to lead productive lives after we are no longer with them. As we help navigate this process, it is important to recognize that some of the pain patients experience may be due to projection of worthwhile parts of the self into the therapist (as discussed in an earlier section of this chapter [see "The Patient's Experience of Termination"]). As we were working through termination, a patient told me, "You bring out what is best in me. I barely recognize who I am when I'm in this room. My mind, my life, even my past and future, all seem full of some new and wonderful meaning. You do this for me....How will I do it alone?" This is a question aligning with early depressive position negotiations. Allowing objects to exist as separate entities is what creates space for the child to do the same for oneself, cultivating an individuality beyond the self-object blurring that characterizes paranoid-schizoid dynamics, in which separateness poses a threat to psychic integrity. In the paranoid-schizoid mindset, one's sense of worth and cohesion will require constant affirmation from external objects, limiting healthy individuation and the ability to learn from experience. If progression from part-object models is not facilitated by early objects, the child's sense of self as a unique, worthwhile individual is stifled. In therapy, we seek to create space for our patients' creative and spontaneous expressions, assigning inherent value to their inner worlds (even if they are completely at odds with our own). Thus, patients can consolidate a sense of self-worth *independent* of anyone else's interpretations of who they are or should be. Part of the sanctity of the frame resides in its *enforcement of separateness*, a necessary component of the therapeutic process. Communing with one's own internal world requires a degree of quietness and solitude. The constant presence of others can impinge on the space for self-reflection. As O'Shaughnessy (1964) stated,

> Absence is a natural and essential condition of a relationship, which otherwise becomes a symbiosis detrimental to the separate identity of either person. Time away from the object is needed to get an emotional perspective on experience had with the object. Appreciation, too, is sharpened in absence. Indeed, the continuous presence of an object would be persecuting;(...)It is not that the child, grudgingly, in the end, tolerates the absent object, but that he has need of its absence. His own emotional growth will help him oppose the forces which make him cling to the object. (pp. 42–43)

Hopefully, as termination is processed in light of the clinical gains garnered over time, patients will reclaim valued aspects of the self that were projected into the therapist. If transitioning to a new provider, patients might feel as though they are starting over and that the progress made thus far will be lost or undone. Yet I do not believe this could *ever* be the case, because something will necessarily have shifted in our patients through continued work. A patient's mind is changed over the course of treatment, as new and unexpected associations are generated, dreams produced, and an immensity of emotionally charged content processed (during and between sessions). If treatment with someone new is initiated, the nature of the work will be quite different, bolstered by the introspection fostered in previous sessions.

While every therapist is undeniably unique, it is our patients' hard work and willingness to be vulnerable that fundamentally drive the therapy forward. After all, we do not provide the overt content for sessions but rather invite anything that is on our patients' minds. We do not tell them what to think or share what *we* have done (or would do) in situations similar to theirs. Rather, therapists serve to model an openness to our patients' internal worlds, encouraging expression beyond the limitations imposed by less receptive figures. It is a new space, full of possibility but approached with suspicion, curiosity, and hope. If our *function* is internalized, patients will increasingly be able to view *themselves* with greater benignity and nuance, furthering self-awareness even when we do not meet. Indeed, this gradual internalization can be appreciated during active treatment, a deepening in the work occurring in tandem with the ability to reconceptualize one's working models of object relationships.

Instances of genuine relatedness and therapeutic progress can help us endure the storms during termination and provide a level of reassurance when things end on a frustrating note. As mentioned earlier, holding this perspective in mind can counterbalance the pull toward identifying as an incompetent, abandoning provider. Thus, patients' attempts to diminish our importance should not be taken at face value. Patients may only be able to process who we are to them when they are not under our gaze or actively defending against grief. Our place in their internal worlds will be shaped and reshaped over time, during treatment and after it has ceased. Accordingly, we cannot expect the significance of our absence to be fully processed while we remain physically *present*. Rather, this dimension will continue to be contemplated well after the therapy has ended. This is to be respected and underlines the kindness in allowing objects their separate existence.

In acknowledging the importance of moments of connectedness, *despite* the transience of the relationship, patients may see worthiness in objects and in themselves beyond part-object constructs. An object need not be possessed or controlled to be of value. If the object leaves, this is not necessarily an indication of the patients' toxic nature or of the insufficiency of their affiliative gestures. Rather, both individuals are respected as whole objects, neither subjectivity impinging on or limiting the dimensionality of the other. Sessions generate an opportunity for two separate minds to grapple with endlessly complex material, achieving deeper insights as thinking becomes a benignly shared endeavor. When the work ends, the value and lessons of the experience will be integrated into the greater arcs of our patients' lives, enriching them yet never defining them. The therapeutic relationship retains its importance *despite* its limitations and finitude. It was never meant to last forever, but there is an eternity to its impact on the lives of both patient and therapist. In reflecting on his work with a patient, Bergstein (2015, pp. 937–938) stated,

> He feels it is momentary and ephemeral, and he wonders whether to surrender to it or whether not to pay too much attention to it since it is temporary anyway.
>
> (…)
>
> I suggest that something in my voice reminded him of a motherly feeling.
>
> He confirms, but immediately adds that he must beware not to get addicted to that feeling.
>
> After some time, he adds: "On second thought, so what if it's just momentary—it's still something."

I will end this section by recounting a dream a patient told me during one of our last sessions together.

> You and I are there. At first, we are on the ground. We're both armed with guns, but neither of us draws. We could have killed each other at any point, I guess.…Yet we don't. We start to build a house together. It becomes a palace, like one of those beautiful ones monarchs live in. We are ascending together, as though we could float, higher and higher as the palace grows taller. We build and build. We stop building and stand on the rooftop. I notice at that point, for the first time, that the palace is made of glass. It's made of glass, but it's so sturdy; I just know it *can't* break. Then the flood comes. Water starts to ascend on the outside of the walls of the palace. I'm feeling desperate, since there's nothing I can do to stop it. I pull out my gun to threaten you, or maybe you pulled out yours first, who can say.…We are both pointing our guns at each other as the water keeps rising, about to engulf us. You look at it, too. You drop your gun and give me a sad smile. I drop mine, too, just as the water swallows both of us. I don't die or wake up.…The water goes away, and I'm on a patch of land.…I'm covered in mud and blood, for some reason. My family is there with me.…We're all huddled together, holding onto each other. Some of them have been dead for a long time, but they're alive, and I don't question it. I'm just happy to be with them. I feel a sense of love and peace beyond anything I have ever felt before. Suddenly I think of you, and at that moment the sun comes out.

Final Reflections

[I]t is joy to be hidden but disaster not to be found.

Donald Winnicott (1963/1965, p. 186)

Throughout this book, I hoped to present how relationships shape our experience of the world. Our sense of self will be established and modified as we connect with others and go through the process of giving them up. Working with patients in psychodynamic therapy can confront us with difficult and unsettling aspects of the human condition, including an awareness of how fragile our lives and relationships are. No matter how jaded or bogged down we become in our profession, we must never forget that our patients are suffering; if we choose to ignore this, our ability to promote healing will be very limited.

The object relations lens is inherently humanistic. It is a model that allows us to seek for that shared, underlying substrate linking all members of our species. Our world seems to revel in creating barriers that relegate certain individuals and groups to a place of fundamental "otherness." If we approach our fellow humans through a lens of intractable misattunement, beyond all reach, we will find ourselves in a social minefield where understanding, reconciliation, mercy, and forgiveness become impossible. Although such divisions may provide a sense of superiority and satisfaction for some, they cause alienation and disconnectedness from the internal world of other humans, which will never be, at its core, entirely distinct from our own. The process of healing entails a giving up of such spurious divisiveness, an acknowledgment of the need to promote an empathic, forgiving stance toward others, recognizing that everyone needs to be valued and loved, for we are all frail, mortal, and fallible. The power of kinship is the guiding light in our quest to recapture our potential for creativity, kindness, and growth. Beyond the factors that divide us, whether visible or invisible, we seek to access the bedrock of common humanity that connects us all. In doing so, we may finally be able to find each other.

KEY POINTS

- The termination process can generate transference and countertransference responses that were less visible during the preceding treatment course. These are fueled by the grieving process taking place in both therapist and patient.

- Patients may react strongly to the impending end, seeking to devalue the therapist or cling to the latter to deny the loss of this important figure.

- These reactions may obscure the therapeutic gains that have taken place until that time. It becomes important for the therapist to hold in mind that the patient's ability to preserve and build on the benefits will remain, even after the treatment is over.

References

Bergstein A: Attacks on linking or a drive to communicate? Tolerating the paradox. Psychoanal Q 84(4):921–942, 2015 26443950

Bion W: Brazilian Lectures: 1973, São Paulo; 1974, Rio de Janeiro/São Paulo. Oxford, UK, Routledge, 1990

Bowlby J: Attachment and Loss, Vol 2: Separation, Anxiety and Anger. London, Hogarth Press and the Institute of Psycho-Analysis, 1973

Boyer LB: Countertransference experiences with severely regressed patients. Contemp Psychoanal 14:48–71, 1978

Ferenczi S: The problem of termination of the analysis (1927), in Final Contributions to the Problems and Methods of Psycho-analysis. Edited by Balint M. London, Karnac, 1994, pp 77–86

Freud S: Observations on transference-love (1915) (Further recommendations on the technique of psycho-analysis III), in The Standard Edition of the Complete Psychological Works of Sigmund Freud, Vol 12. Translated and edited by Strachey J. London, Hogarth Press, 1953, pp 157–171

Freud S: Mourning and melancholia (1917[1915]), in The Standard Edition of the Complete Psychological Works of Sigmund Freud, Vol 14. Translated and edited by Strachey J. London, Hogarth Press, 1957, pp 109–140

Freud S: New introductory lectures on psycho-analysis (1933[1932]), in The Standard Edition of the Complete Psychological Works of Sigmund Freud, Vol 22. Translated and edited by Strachey J. London, Hogarth Press, 1964, pp 1–182

Freud S: Analysis terminable and interminable (1937), in The Standard Edition of the Complete Psychological Works of Sigmund Freud, Vol 23. Translated and edited by Strachey J. London, Hogarth Press, 1964, pp 209–254

Gabbard GO: What is a "good enough" termination? J Am Psychoanal Assoc 57(3):575–594, 2009 19620466

Klein M: Notes on some schizoid mechanisms. Int J Psychoanal 27 (Pt 3–4):99–110, 1946 20261821

Klein M: On the criteria for the termination of a psycho-analysis. Int J Psychoanal 31:78–80, 1950

Lafarge L: Termination and repetition: the dissolution of the frame. Int J Psychoanal 100(6):1270–1285, 2019 33945738

Lichtenberg JD: Experience as a guide to psychoanalytic theory and practice. J Am Psychoanal Assoc 46(1):16–36, discussion 36–84, 1998 9565899

Lussana S: Termination of a psychoanalysis: some notes on theory, technique, and clinical material. Int J Psychoanal 99(3):603–626, 2018 33951808

Orens MH: Setting a termination date, an impetus to analysis. J Am Psychoanal Assoc 3(4):651–665, 1955 13271223

Orgel S: Letting go: some thoughts about termination. J Am Psychoanal Assoc 48(3):719–738, 2000 11059394

O'Shaughnessy E: The absent object. J Child Psychother 1:34–43, 1964

Steiner J: The equilibrium between the paranoid-schizoid and the depressive positions. New Library of Psychoanalysis 14:46–58, 1992

Winnicott DW: Communicating and not communicating leading to a study of certain opposites (1963), in The Maturational Processes and the Facilitating Environment. Edited by Khan M. London, Hogarth Press and the Institute of Psycho-Analysis, 1965, pp 179–192

Winnicott DW: The use of an object. Int J Psychoanal 50:711–716, 1969

Index

Entries followed by a lower-case *n* and a number (i.e., *14n9*) indicate material contained in footnotes and the number of the specific footnote.